PATIENT
IN THE
WOMB

PATIENT
IN THE
WOMB

by

E. Peter Volpe

MERCER

Patient in the Womb
Copyright © 1984
Mercer University Press, Macon GA 31207
All rights reserved
Printed in the United States of America

All books published by Mercer University Press
are produced on acid-free paper that exceeds
the minimum standards set by the National
Historical Publications and Records Commission.

Library of Congress Cataloging in Publication Data
Volpe, E. Peter (Erminio Peter)
Patient in the womb.
Includes bibliographical references and index.
1. Fetus—Diseases—Genetic aspects.   2. Fetus—
Abnormalities.   3. Prenatal diagnosis.   I. Title.
RG626.V6   1984   618.3   84-10746
ISBN 0-86554-122-1 (alk. paper)

CONTENTS

LIST OF PLATES

PREFACE

The expectant mother is inherently apprehensive, but no feeling is more pervasive than the fear of giving birth to a deformed child. A concrete expression of this fear is the question so often asked immediately following delivery: "Is my baby normal?" Universally, the mother's first look at her newborn infant is anxious and searching.

Defects at birth that doom the infant to an early death or a lifetime of illness take an enormous toll in human life and potential. A deformed child is delivered into the world every thirty seconds. No statistic, however, can speak for the psychological trauma suffered by the parents. The birth of a malformed child imposes an emotional burden on the parents to which adjustment is slow and agonizing. It is difficult for parents to wash away the deep anxieties and unjustified feelings of guilt or shame that they experience. In affluent societies, ours included, birth defects still loom as one of our serious problems.

Advances in the medical sciences in recent years have been truly awesome. Technologies have been developed that have extended life to many high-risk newborn infants who, in an earlier era, would have quickly perished. Medical progress has been so extraordinary that some fetal malformations can now be treated *before* the fetus is delivered. Clearly, the human fetus has attained the status of a patient. The advent of fetal therapy raises visions of either medical miracles or brave new worlds, depending on one's point of view.

Medicine has become more than a comfort-and-care profession. It is a major scientific discipline with the capabilities of profoundly affecting human life. Each new medical success provides potential for both opportunities and for perils. The remarkable advances have raised a whole spectrum of ethical, social, and legal dilemmas that present acute challenges to existing moral codes and conventional wisdom.

With the growing awareness of the new medical technologies, the public is eager to learn of the new knowledge. However, much of the information appears in technical journals not readily accessible to, nor easily understood by, the interested layperson. While this book should appeal to health professionals, it was not written primarily for them. It has been prepared for the general reader who is trained neither in medicine nor genetics. It differs from many scientific books on prenatal diagnosis in that it draws the reader's attention to complex moral, social, and legal problems. To many specialists, it may seem that I have frequently stated the obvious; to the generalist it may appear that on occasion I have dwelled on too much detail. It is my hope that accuracy has not been compromised in the attempt to present a clear, concise account of the present state of knowledge of congenital defects, and the promises and threats of the new medical technologies.

I have benefited from enjoyable and spirited discussions I have had with my colleagues at the Mercer University School of Medicine. Several colleagues, notably Dr. Charles Hockman, meticulously reviewed various chapters and provided constructive criticism. I have been fortunate in having the patient and untiring assistance of Wilma Parrish, research associate at the Mercer Medical School. I am grateful to Carolyn T. Volpe, biomedical illustrator at the medical school, who prepared the drawings with her usual expertise and care. Ms. India Fuller of the Mercer University Press offered many valuable suggestions that have made the contents more readable.

Mercer University
School of Medicine

E. Peter Volpe
Professor of Basic
Medical Sciences

Fall 1983

CHAPTER I

QUALITY OF LIFE

I n the fall of 1963, a baby born to a couple in a Baltimore hospital was diagnosed as having Down syndrome.[1] This congenital disorder, misleadingly labeled "mongolism," was indelibly stamped on the child's face: a prominent forehead, a flat nasal bridge, a chronically open mouth, a projecting lower lip, a large protruding tongue, and slanting eyes (Plate I). The infant also suffered from duodenal atresia, an intes-

---

[1]In 1886, Dr. John Langdon Down (1828-1896), a London physician, provided the first comprehensive description of a puzzling type of congenital mental retardation. He unjustifiably seized upon the Oriental-like cast of the eyes of the affected newborn to designate the condition as "mongolism" or "mongoloid idiocy." Down's theory was that the anomaly represented a regression to an earlier and more primitive human form analogous to Mongolian peoples. Down's peculiar ethnic viewpoint is, of course, untenable and the labels of "mongoloid idiot" and "mongol" are being discarded in scientific literature and popular press. It deserves emphasis that affected children bear no true resemblance to Mongolian peoples (unless they happen to be born among them). The eyefolds of the afflicted child only superficially resemble the characteristic folds of Oriental persons. Medical scientists today have proposed to call the disorder "Down syndrome," a term that has gained acceptance and use. Current convention dictates the modified term, "Down syndrome," rather than "Down's syndrome."

tinal obstruction that precludes the intake of food by mouth. The blockage is correctable without difficulty by an operation of nominal risk.

The attending physicians kept the infant alive by intravenous feeding and made arrangements for remedial intestinal surgery. However, consent to the surgical intervention was denied by the parents, who wished their malformed child to have a reprieve from what they perceived would be pointless future suffering. The medical staff of the hospital acceded to the parents' request, tempering efforts to seek a court order to override the parents' decision. In the absence of surgery to remedy the intestinal obstruction, the infant died of starvation in the hospital on the eleventh day.[2]

In ancient Greek and Roman times, malformed babies were left either to perish from exposure in the mountains or cast into the rivers and seas. Infanticide, taking the life of a sickly infant, was then a common practice. Today, we view with repugnance the primitive procedure of abandonment of the sickly infant. Yet in the absence of prenatal diagnosis of a severe deformity, it is only at birth that a gross malformation becomes glaringly observable. The birth of a retarded child with multiple body deformities creates a grievous crisis for the parents, especially if the life of the child will almost certainly be one of excessive hardship. Is it morally permissible to end in compassion a life that is undeniably destined to be burdensome, with the expectation that a better new life may be conceived in a subsequent pregnancy? Opinions and consciences are greatly divided on this sensitive issue.

The newborn is obviously incapable of self-determination. The malformed infant is unable to judge whether its existence will be severely compromised. Others must decide whether the child's life will be marginal or futile.[3] Who has the responsibility to act on behalf of the ab-

---

[2]This case is not an isolated one. On 14 April 1982, a six-day-old infant died at a hospital in Bloomington, Indiana, after his parents denied him routine surgery to correct a tracheo-esophageal fistula, a condition in which the esophagus is not connected to the stomach. In this instance, a lower court upheld their decision. See N. Fost, "Legislating morality: The Bloomington baby and section 504," *Hastings Center Report* 12 (1982): 5-8.

[3]Given the impossibility of gaining the consent of the newborn patient to withhold treatment on itself, one might argue that the life of the newborn must be prolonged until the patient develops decision-making capabilities in later years. Ironically, this might prompt an unusual type of legal action: a suit for wrongful life. Children have brought

normal newborn? Does the burden of decision making fall on the parents? Are physicians justified in making value judgments under the guise of a medical decision? What are the legal ramifications?

Medical accomplishments in recent years have been extraordinary. The powers of modern science have become both novel and awe-inspiring. Progress in medical research has occurred too rapidly to permit the average person to digest the rush of recent discoveries. The brisk output of new knowledge disturbs one's serenity.[4] Moreover, the remarkable discoveries have created value problems where none existed before. It is much easier to live in a society with fixed values or a universal moral standard than to live in a society that is constantly changing. The old certainty of our values has been threatened.

Society remains bridled by dogmas that trace their origin to a period in time when our early ancestors were awed by nature and mystified by life itself. Such mysticism and wonder have declined with increasing knowledge and understanding. Each medical innovation is rooted in new knowledge and is accompanied by a fresh outlook. Too often, however, the newer information is distorted to conform to preexisting patterns of attitudes, beliefs, and actions. It would suggest that adjustments in values have to be made when new knowledge in a changing situation does not reinforce values based on a different set of circumstances.

Modern medicine has ingeniously developed technologies that prolong the lives of many high-risk infants who, in an earlier time, would have had little chance for survival. When techniques did not exist to keep high-risk infants alive, there were no heart-searching decisions to make. It bears emphasizing that the acute challenges to existing moral codes have stemmed from the successes of modern medicine, not the failures. With each success, one additional type of congenital malformation has

---

suit against their parents seeking to recover damages for physical handicaps inextricably tied to their birth (for example, congenital deformities, congenital syphilis, illegitimacy). In some of the cases, the courts have recognized the justice of the child's claim of injury due to parental negligence.

[4]The lay public views the awesome advances of science with considerable suspicious concern and hostility, a factor that has been noted by writers as diverse as John D. Erskine in his *The Moral Obligation to be Intelligent, and Other Essays* (Freeport: Books for Libraries Press, 1969) and Richard Hofstadter, *Anti-intellectualism in American Life* (New York: Alfred A. Knopf and Company, 1970).

been removed from the "unsalvageable" category of past years.[5] Strong voices have now been raised as to whether the prolongation of life is of clear benefit to each and every child. We can no longer eschew certain incisive questions. What kind of life are we saving? Are we inexorably constrained by theistic philosophy and medical idealism that all life must be saved at any cost? Are we prepared, prompted by humanitarian considerations, to make an exception to the time-honored ethic based on the "sanctity of life" and endorse, in particular instances, a guiding principle that embraces the "quality of life"?[6]

Death as a result of withholding medical care constitutes a significant proportion of neonatal deaths.[7] The usual practice of allowing the death of anencephalic infants—those who congenitally lack all or most of the brain—can be understood as a decision based on the absence of any possibility of these infants achieving a minimal degree of human activity or social interaction. A slow, painful death is a certainty for a child born with an irreversible neurologic deficit, such as severe myelomeningocele (open spinal cord).[8] These are conditions that are profoundly

---

[5]As a result of the relentless pursuit to save the lives of more and more infants, the United States has enjoyed a 58 percent decrease in infant death rate in the short span of 30 years. The reduction is related in large measure to the application of new knowledge to the care of infants. See M. E. Wegman, "Annual summary of vital statistics—1970," *Pediatrics* 48 (1971): 979-83.

[6]The validity of the commandment, "Thou Shalt Not Kill," as a universal rule is not contested here. We should acknowledge, however, that society does examine the justness of the rule in special circumstances and occasionally permits an exception, such as the sanction of capital punishment. Our purpose here is to explore whether allowing a severely defective newborn to die represents justifiably another special exception to the third commandment.

[7]In one special-care nursery in a university medical center over a two-year period, treatment was withheld in one out of ten newborn infants, whose prognosis for meaningful life was judged to be poor or hopeless. See R. S. Duff and A. G. M. Campbell, "Moral and ethical dilemmas in the special-care nursery," *New England Journal of Medicine* 289 (1973): 890-94.

[8]There were no options available to physicians when myelomeningocele (open spina bifida) was untreatable. Beginning with new surgical procedures in the early 1960s, the tendency has been to vigorously treat all infants with this condition. The surgical treatment, however, is not always an unqualified success. Some spina bifida children who are saved by surgery are paralyzed and incontinent for the rest of their lives, and may be mentally retarded. Modern treatment has greatly increased the prospect of survival, but that survival may mean a life of such gross handicap that the justification for treatment is often questioned.

incompatible with a meaningful existence. Those who oppose the hastening of death of a newborn with Down syndrome point out that this anomaly does not exclude all capacity for normal human satisfactions. Who decides when life is not worth living? Broad support can be marshaled for the view that the decision-making process is highly personal, revolving around the emotional resources of the parents faced with the lifetime sentence of a child with severe defects. The parents are the ones who must live with, and are most affected by, their decision.

A diagnosis of Down syndrome invariably affects the parents deeply. As with any serious diagnosis, the parents can expect to experience a range of emotions, some even frightening and contradictory. The mother in the Baltimore hospital grieved when she learned of her child's infirmity. After the initial stage of shock and disbelief, the mother reconciled the situation emotionally and carefully examined the long-term prognosis for her child.[9] In her eyes, the child's incurable affliction and lifelong dependency, along with the emotional and economic trauma to the family, justified for her the willful termination of the life of her child. The husband shared his wife's feeling that it would be unfair to inflict the burden of a retarded child on their other children. The attending physicians attempted to alleviate the parents' anxieties by stressing that mental retardation admits of degree. The genetic imbalance[10] that causes Down syndrome allows for wide variation in mental abilities, be-

---

[9]Down syndrome may not be immediately apparent to the parents and unless specifically informed, they may believe that their child is normal. Most studies urge that the parents be told as soon as a definite diagnosis has been made. It is now customary to confirm the clinical diagnosis by chromosomal analysis. See J. Carr, "Mongolism: Telling the parents," *Developmental Medicine and Child Neurology* 12 (1970): 213-21; and P. Pinkerton, "Parental acceptance of the handicapped child," ibid., 207-12.

[10]For a long time, medical opinion erred grievously in recognizing the true cause of Down syndrome. At one time or another, syphilis, tuberculosis, malnutrition, thyroid deficiency, emotional shock, and even alcoholism were incriminated as causes of mongolism. In 1959, the young pediatrician Jérôme Lejeune and his colleagues, Marthe Gautier and Raymond Turpin, at the University of Paris studied the chromosomes of cells taken from the skin of infants with Down syndrome. They employed the newly discovered technique of culturing skin cells and preparing them for chromosome analysis. It came as a curious surprise when the team found that the cells of affected children do not contain the normal chromosome number of 46, but rather 47. The additional chromosome was one of the very small chromosomes, but this slight excess of genetic material was sufficient to disrupt the normal developmental processes and affect many different parts of the body (see chapter 2).

havior, and developmental progress. Nevertheless, one cannot overlook the constant adjustments and formidable difficulties in parenting a Down child.

Physicians have an ingrained obligation to preserve life and to maximize the infant's potential, however limited it may be. In their customary approach to patients, physicians habitually pull from their therapeutic armamentarium an antibiotic or drug that checks or reverses the course of a disease. The vast majority of diseases are infectious and treatable. The damage of an inheritable disorder, however, is usually irreversible. In most genetic defects, medical treatment is simply palliative, if not wholly ineffectual. Even in the face of the most efficacious therapeutic manipulations, the Down child can never enjoy the satisfactions of intellectual or physical achievement known to a normal person. Clearly, if the child had not been handicapped by Down syndrome, the physicians would have undoubtedly corrected the duodenal atresia. It is fair to say that the attending physicians were motivated by compassion[11] as well as an overall respect for the judgments of the parents. A nationwide survey of the attitudes of pediatricians and pediatric surgeons disclosed that two-thirds of them would acquiesce to a parental request to withhold treatment of duodenal atresia in a Down child.[12]

Not all physicians perceive their responsibility as limited solely to presenting parents with the necessary information to permit informed decisions.[13] Some contend that the onus of decision making falls on the

---

[11]Even traditional-minded philosophers will admit that compassionate or kindly acts are, at the very least, virtuous. Such a praiseworthy outlook offers scant consolation to the American Association on Mental Deficiency, an organization that views the blatant failure of surgical intervention as a threat to the right to life of mentally retarded persons. In a position paper in 1973, the association stated: "It is our position that the existence of mental retardation is no justification for the terminating of the life of any human being or for permitting such a life to be terminated either directly or through the withholding of life sustaining procedures." See D. Smith, "Down's syndrome, amniocentesis, and abortion: Prevention or elimination?" *Mental Retardation* 19 (1981): 8-11.

[12]A. Shaw, J. G. Randolph, and B. Manard, "Ethical issues in pediatric surgery: A national survey of pediatricians and pediatric surgeons," *Pediatrics* 60 (1977): 588-99.

[13]A fervent minority of physicians have expressed concern about the inadequacy of medical treatment of newborn infants with birth defects. See R. E. Cooke, "Whose suffering?" *Journal of Pediatrics* 80 (1972): 906-908; F. J. Ingelfinger, "Bedside ethics for the hopeless case," *New England Journal of Medicine* 289 (1973): 914-15; N. Fost, "Passive euthanasia of patients with Down's syndrome," *Archives of Internal Medicine* 142

physician in whose care the child has been placed. Others assert that the death of an untreated infant is an unacceptable means of alleviating suffering. Still others urge that other alternatives should be explored or offered, such as adoption, which is often available for children with Down syndrome. Several have expressed concern that the "eliminative" approach to Down syndrome encourages a retrenchment from the search for ameliorative measures and therapeutic innovations. This group contends that it could well signal the abandonment of the investment of both creative thought and funds in special education and training. Differing opinions of this sort are inevitable in a situation that involves value choices rather than technical expertise. Nevertheless, a professional who is an expert in technical matters should not be thought of as having special competence in decision making that relates to resolving an ethical issue.

The courts have provided little guidance on this complex problem. In cases involving older children with life-threatening illnesses, judges have overruled the parents and have ordered lifesaving measures such as blood transfusions. The therapeutic procedures usually restore the child to a normal existence. The correction of duodenal atresia, however, provides little relief from the multiple debilities of a Down child. Legal precedent involving the withholding of essential treatment from a congenitally incapacitated infant is meager. Theoretically, criminal liability on the grounds of homicide by omission or child neglect is possible, but parents and physicians have rarely been prosecuted for withholding care from defective neonates. The legality of the practice or the appropriateness of current law is not likely to be ignored indefinitely.[14]

As more cases of withholding medical treatment surface and gain visibility, there will doubtlessly be heightened public concern and outrage.[15] Any public discussion of the delicate moral issues would quickly

---

(1982): 2295; and Smith, "Down's syndrome, amniocentesis, and abortion: Prevention or elimination?"

[14]The possible legal liabilities for the willful termination of life of the newborn are aptly discussed by J. A. Robertson and N. Fost, "Passive euthanasia of defective newborn infants: Legal consideration," *Journal of Pediatrics* 88 (1976): 888-89.

[15]There is a tendency in society to look at an ethical viewpoint from the "wedge" concept or "camel's head" argument, which asserts that to permit one action opens the door, or tent, to another, even more offensive, action. Thus, this argument contends that acceptance of the termination of life of a Down child will lead inevitably to the wholesale

deteriorate into slogans such as "life must be preserved at all cost" or "what right have physicians to play God?"[16] Witness, for example, the recurrent ideological battle cries in the anxiety-ridden public and legislative debate on abortion. It is futile to expect the different segments of a pluralistic society to reach a consensus on a sensitive issue. When there are irreconcilable differences on issues of morality, legislative bodies enact into law one set of beliefs and impose them on those who conscientiously believe otherwise. Like so many other attempts at legislating morality, more distress is usually created than is relieved.

Some have argued for increasing the involvement of the courts in decisions concerning life and death, on the grounds that the disinterested or dispassionate courts, unlike parents and physicians, have no vested interest in the outcome. There are, however, a number of compelling arguments against establishing a law that would prescribe the standards by which the withholding of lifesaving care for seriously ill infants is legally permissible. The most conspicuous problem would be the extreme difficulty of formulating criteria to distinguish between justified and unjustified deaths. It is unlikely that the law would grant broad discretion to the parents, physicians, or hospital authorities. The expectation from any new legislation would be that the authorization to terminate life be restricted only to infants who are "tragically deformed." We would then be faced with the decision of which cases fit precisely the narrow legislative description of malformation. The decision, once again, would call for value judgment. Consensus on withholding treatment would be relatively easy in the extreme case of very mild abnormalities or very severe abnormalities, but exceedingly agonizing in the vast and ill-defined gray zone. No court is likely to approve the withholding of routine care from an infant with a club foot or cleft lip, or to intervene when an anencephalic child is allowed to die without intensive care or surgery. But con-

---

termination of the life of a child with a very minor deformity, such as a cleft lip. Such an emotive concept is unimpressive. An ethical principle is valid only over a certain limited range; when pushed outside its limit, the principle tends to become absurd. Even Oliver Wendell Holmes could not extend the principle of free speech to those who falsely cried "fire" in a crowded theatre.

[16] If the phrase "playing God" means interfering with nature, then medical scientists have "played God" for many decades. Virtually every newborn is the beneficiary of some meddling with nature, whether it be heating the nursery, placing silver nitrate drops in the eyes, feeding through a synthetic nipple, or using a mechanical respirator.

sensus is lost when abnormalities such as Down syndrome and spina bifida are involved.[17]

The morality of allowing a malformed infant to die is a matter not easily laid to rest. At present, much latitude in decision making has been tolerated. Physicians appear to have a strong preference for limiting decision making to the parent-physician partnership, as well as a strong bias against subjecting the problem to review and resolution by committees or courts. In turn, the parents have not been reluctant to bear the burden of decision making. In the foregoing case, the parents did not feel that they committed a great moral wrong. Was it morally reprehensible?

James Gustafson, professor of theological ethics at the University of Chicago, finds their decision morally repugnant.[18] Gustafson does not view the Down infant as presenting a clear threat to family integration. He submits that raising a retarded child does not present intolerable and unbearable suffering to the mother, father, or the rest of the family.[19] Moreover, he sees the Down infant as being capable of responding to love and of being trainable to accept responsibilities within his or her restricted capacities. John Robertson, a professor of law at the University

---

[17]Allowing a severely defective infant to die is often identified as passive euthanasia (for example, withholding or withdrawing means of life support), in contrast to active euthanasia (such as administering a lethal dose). Passive euthanasia generally receives less opposition than active euthanasia. However, James Rachels ("Active and passive euthanasia," *New England Journal of Medicine* 292 [1975]: 78-80) argues that active euthanasia is, in many cases, more humane than passive euthanasia. If one simply withholds treatment, Rachels states, it may take the patient longer to die, and the patient may suffer more than if a quick and relatively painless lethal injection had been administered.

[18]J. M. Gustafson, "Mongolism, parental desires, and the right to life," *Perspectives in Biology and Medicine* 16 (1973): 529-57. See also P. Ramsey, *The Patient as Person* (New Haven: Yale University Press, 1970).

[19]Propositions that "suffering is endurable" or "suffering is ennobling" are products of armchair exercise and idealism. Should we knowingly add suffering to our lives? Clearly, living with the handicapped is a family affair, and only the members of a family can determine the limits of suffering that they can bear. Yet, one may find comforting the remarks of Pearl Buck, the mother of a child retarded by phenylketonuria: "A retarded child, a handicapped person, brings its own gift to life, even to the life of a normal human being. That gift is comprehended in the lessons of patience, understanding, and mercy, lessons which we all need to receive and to practice with one another, whatever we are." P. S. Buck, "Foreword," *The Terrible Choice: The Abortion Dilemma* (New York: Bantam Books, 1968) ix-xi.

of Wisconsin, defends Gustafson's views by declaring that life is preferable to death even when that life is accompanied by impairment or suffering.[20]

On the other hand, Joseph Fletcher, a Christian ethicist at the University of Virginia Medical School, believes that every infant is entitled to a reasonable chance of achieving what he calls "humanhood." By humanhood, Fletcher means a state that includes self-awareness, a sense of futurity, and the ability to relate to others.[21] Richard McCormick, a moral theologian, concurs that life is not a value to be preserved in and for itself.[22] He states that life is a value to be preserved only insofar as it contains some potential for human relationships. Accordingly, biological life in itself is neither sacrosanct nor intrinsically good; there are more valuable aspects than merely being alive.

The moral issues are difficult and complex. The mother of the Down infant raised a moral question when she asked: What ought I do? The conservative and absolutist attitudes of Gustafson and the liberal tenets of Fletcher exemplify two basically different views of morality. Within one view, moral rules constitute commands that must be obeyed as absolute standards. Moral goodness is thought to lie in conformity to rules for their own sake. The validity of the rules is in no way dependent on the good or bad consequences of obedience. This form of morality is deeply rooted in Judeo-Christian religion. The absolute standards are the same for all people regardless of time, place, and circumstances. Under such sanctions, to contrive the termination of life of a Down infant is morally wrong.[23]

---

[20]J. A. Robertson, "Involuntary euthanasia of defective newborns," *Stanford Law Review* 27 (1975): 213-14, 251-61.

[21]J. Fletcher, *Morals and Medicine* (Boston: Beacon Press, 1960) and *The Ethics of Genetic Control* (Garden City: Doubleday, Anchor Press, 1974).

[22]R. A. McCormick, "To save or let die: The dilemma of modern medicine," *Journal of the American Medical Association* 229 (1974): 172-76.

[23]A long tradition of religious, philosophical, and legal thought and action holds that life is to be preserved, even at great cost. Every moment of human life is considered intrinsically sacred. According to Roman Catholic moral theology, the right to life of a human being derives not from the parents or from society but directly from God. Christian morality views the taking of life as an immoral act that violates God's law. The strong religious ideals contribute to sustaining our system of legal sanctions and make the taking of human life a source of guilt and anxiety.

Within the second context of morality, moral rules are subordinate to consequences. Moral principles exist solely for achieving certain ends and are to be judged by their tendency to promote those ends. Those who support this position generally state that moral rules are to be judged by their tendency to promote or maximize human happiness. Accordingly, the issue of terminating the life of a Down newborn cannot be resolved by appeals to self-evident moral principles. There are no absolute answers to questions about life. An individual who subscribes to this approach makes decisions in the light of new knowledge and experience.[24]

At first glance, a thorny ethical problem seems to have been resolved by a surprisingly simple solution—freedom for each person to act as he or she believes right. Each individual establishes his or her own morality. Ethics becomes simply the dictates of individual conscience.[25] There can be little doubt that we have witnessed the end of a monistic society and the emergence of a pluralistic society, at least in the West. In a pluralistic society, by definition, there cannot be a single set of values, ends, meanings, and purposes. The old equation of rightness and custom breaks down. Pluralism entitles individuals to hold and be respected for their views.[26]

---

[24]The two views of morality presented here represent the two basic, and mutually exclusive, ethical tenets that have received the most attention in recent years: teleological and deontological. The teleological attitude assesses the worth of actions by their consequences; in contrast, the deontological approach maintains that the rightness or wrongness of human action is independent of ends and consequences. Thus, the teleological concept denies precisely what the deontological view affirms. For additional details, see T. L. Beauchamp and J. F. Childress, *Principles of Biomedical Ethics* (New York: Oxford University Press, 1979); T. A. Mappes and J. S. Zembety, *Biomedical Ethics* (New York: McGraw-Hill Book Company, 1981).

[25]Is it simply enough to say that the only ethical requirement is that each person establish his or her own morality? According to several philosophers, advocates of free choice ignore a fundamental proposition. The refusal to regulate by a universal moral code merely postpones the day when some collective judgment will be required. Moral rules are necessary because one person's aims in life often conflict with the aims of others. They are useful in restraining a person from doing things that affect the freedom of others adversely. It would be ideal if each of us could pursue our own ends without thwarting other people in the pursuit of theirs. More often than not, however, the actions of one person do have perceptible effects on other people. Hence, some philosophers contend that the search for a new ethic must begin with the view that moral propositions are societal, not individual, matters.

[26]A utilitarian theory known as "situation ethics" has been advocated by Joseph

When reasonable and rational people disagree about whether an infant's future is clouded by a severe deformity, it would seem that the parents are best situated to make the final judgment. In order to balance alternative consequences, the parents should be as fully informed as possible about the nature of the congenital abnormality. They then can evaluate carefully. What are the relevant facts in Down syndrome? What do we know about the development and maturation of a Down infant? What is the level of intelligence and degree of educability of the Down child? What special education and training assistance is available? What are the serious health problems?

The most serious, irreversible complication is the state of mental retardation that occurs in every child with Down syndrome. The mental age typically attained at maturity is between three and seven years of age.[27] This means that Down individuals usually function at intellectual levels no higher than that of a seven-year-old. They are educable but learn very slowly.[28] Less than four in 100 are able to read with comprehension; only two in 100 ever learn to write. Many Down children appear brighter than they are because of their cheerful and gregarious disposition. Much of their learning is accomplished by imitation as they generally have strong powers of mimicry. Although sociable and good-

---

Fletcher, *Situation Ethics: The New Morality* (Philadelphia: Westminster Press, 1963). In this type of moral philosophy, the conscience ranges free in response to concrete reasons. Each situation is seen as being different and even unique, and no general rules can possibly be of much help in dealing with the dynamics of a concrete situation. There are no criteria or guiding principles for determining what is right or wrong in particular cases. The method involves becoming clear about the facts in the case and then forming a judgment about what is to be done. Briefly, situation ethics states that the variables in a given case determine what one ought to do. A given decision is not intrinsically or invariably good or evil. The rightness or propriety of an action or decision depends on the situation.

[27]The administration of standardized "intelligence" tests is difficult because of the short attention span and poor muscular coordination of the Down child. Generally, children with Down syndrome have IQ scores between 20 and 50; some attain scores in the 60s and 70s.

[28]The prognosis for intellectual development of the Down child is currently being reevaluated. Recent studies indicate that the educability of Down children has been underestimated, even in informed professional circles. See J. E. Rynders, D. Spiker, and J. M. Horrobin, "Underestimating the educability of Down's syndrome children: Examination of methodological problems in recent literature," *American Journal of Mental Deficiency* 82 (1978): 440-48.

natured, Down children tend to be stubborn. The poor muscle tone of children with Down syndrome interferes with physical development and activities. The affected infant is late in sitting, crawling, and walking. Whereas normal infants begin to walk at the age of 12 months, most infants with Down syndrome do not learn to walk until two to three years of age. Their movements remain slow and clumsy throughout life.

The Down person cannot manage his or her own affairs and must always remain dependent on others. Affected individuals account for about 15 percent of the inmates of institutions for mental defectives in the United States.[29] In the past, many affected newborns were placed in mental institutions within a week of diagnosis, a practice that has clearly dwindled. Down children living at home are superior in both social and physical development to those confined at birth in institutions. They are more educable, are taller, and walk at an earlier age than those institutionalized shortly after birth.

In recent years, an increasing number of programs have become available to inform parents of learning experiences for their Down infant. These children benefit from sensory stimulation programs that are initiated in the first few months of life. They are encouraged to engage in specific exercises involving both gross and fine motor activities. The teaching of self-help skills (including feeding, toilet training, and dressing) allows the child to function more independently.

Down children are beset with numerous health problems. Heart lesions are common, accounting for one-third of the deaths that occur during the first year of life. The children are also especially vulnerable to bacterial and viral infections. In the past, acute lung infections (pneumonia) and intestinal infections (gastroenteritis) were the major causes

---

[29]The discussion here has excluded the utilitarian consideration of the financial burden—to the family and society—of caring for a severely defective child. Nonetheless, the cost of caring for a Down person is not an entirely irrelevant factor. In the United States, almost all Down patients are institutionalized sooner or later. It is estimated that one-third are institutionalized in infancy, one-third around age 10, and one-third around age 30. For the average patient, the remaining years of care in an institution cost conservatively about $60,000. In one county alone in Georgia (DeKalb County), of approximately 6,500 births per year, eight children are born with Down syndrome. The incidence is 1.2 per 1,000 live births, which is not significantly different from the usual reported incidence of 1.0 per 1,000. Conservatively, in the state of Georgia alone, care for a minimum of 30 Down children born in one year from pregnancies in women 35 or older costs the state at least $1,800,000.

of death. Today, however, life expectancy has been increased dramatically by the widespread use of antibiotics. At birth, the life expectancy is 16 years. However, for those who survive the most critical first year of life, the expectation increases to 40 years.

People with Down syndrome have a varied assortment of other defects. The neck is typically short and broad; the skin is rosy but rough and dry; the teeth are abnormally shaped and irregularly aligned; and the gonads and genitalia are underdeveloped. Among males, beard and pubic growth are scant. The males who survive to reproductive age are sterile; there is no known case of a male with Down syndrome fathering children. Females with Down syndrome have fared better; at least a dozen affected females with offspring have been recorded. Since the vast majority never reproduce, affected children nearly always come from normal parents.

There are many unusual features of the hands of Down patients. Typically broad and stumpy, the hands are from 10 to 30 percent shorter than normal hands. In particular, the fifth, or "little," finger is unusually small and incurved (Plate I). The dermatoglyphic, or ridge, patterns of the fingers, palms, and soles are grossly abnormal. On the finger tips, the dermal ridges are arranged primarily in loops; normal patterns such as whorls and arches are greatly reduced in number. The palm of the hand has a prominent single transverse fold or crease, the so-called "simian line." In normal individuals, there are usually two lines (rather than one straight line) across the upper part of the palm. The feet of a Down child, often short and clumsy, have a characteristic well-marked gap between the first and second toe (Plate I).

About four percent of Down babies are born with incomplete development of the intestine. There are several areas in which the intestinal tract can fail to develop properly. There can be an obstruction in the tube (esophagus) leading to the stomach or, more frequently, a blockage just beyond the stomach in the small intestine (duodenum). The last part of the bowel may be unable to function (Hirschsprung's disease). Leukemia, an uncontrolled growth of white blood cells, is about ten times more common in Down subjects than in normal children.

Notwithstanding their outward congenial disposition, serious behavioral problems are not uncommon in Down children. It is difficult to determine the origin of the behavioral problems. Some of the problems may be due to an insecure home environment, while others may be caused by the stresses of coping with the pressures of life in a "normal" world. Down adults age prematurely. In middle age, there is a strong tendency for many Down patients to withdraw, become demented, and develop the pathologic changes associated with Alzheimer's disease. This disease is characterized by the deterioration of speech and communication and is accompanied by a profound loss of memory.

Clearly, the Down infant can reach a point of significant fulfillment of his or her limited potentials—given proper and constant care. The Down infant has the capacity to love and be loved, and can acquire a feeling of self-worth. However, the mental level is typically very low, with emotional development and general behavior fixed at a childhood level. The Down child is heavily dependent on attention and approval. The affected child suffers from several very serious physical ailments that severely impact on his or her activities.

CHAPTER II

PRENATAL DIAGNOSIS

U ntil recently, pediatricians were limited in their capacity to determine if an expectant mother might deliver a child with a serious birth defect. For the most part, pediatricians referred prospective parents with a family history of some congenital disorder to specialists in genetic counseling. Even then the prospective parents could be informed only of the statistical probability that they would have a child with a particular congenital disorder. No assurance could be given that the actual outcome of the pregnancy would not be unfavorable. Many high-risk couples in the past avoided pregnancy rather than hazard the birth of a defective child. Today, this situation has been altered dramatically by the availability of techniques that reveal a disorder while the fetus is still developing in the mother. This new approach to the detection of genetic diseases is referred to as "prenatal diagnosis."

The purpose of prenatal diagnosis is to identify abnormalities in infants prior to birth. The rationale for preventing genetic defects is to reduce human suffering. It bears repeating that the thrust of prenatal diagnosis is to prevent the tragic impact of serious genetic diseases, and not to manipulate or "engineer" the genetic makeup of an individual.

Another aspect of prenatal diagnosis is that it is undertaken only with voluntary participation and informed consent.

A number of inherited disorders can be diagnosed *in utero* by a procedure known as amniocentesis, which involves the removal of a sample of the fluid in the amniotic cavity surrounding the developing fetus.[1] Cells are continually shed into the amniotic fluid and these free-floating cells have been shown to be of fetal origin. They can be grown in laboratory culture to preview the chromosomes and enzymes of the fetus (Plate II). Amniocentesis is not performed frivolously or prompted by idle curiosity. The technique is no longer novel or experimental.[2] At the outset, it is important to identify pregnancies appropriate for this type of examination. Stated another way, there must be good reason to expect the possibility of the presence of a serious congenital defect. Furthermore, the defect must be one that is susceptible to diagnosis from the cells or fluids that are obtained by amniocentesis.

A clear-cut warrant for amniocentesis is the increased risk in older women of producing children with Down syndrome. This congenital disorder is most common in the offspring of women over 35 and particularly over 40 years of age. In many clinics today, amniocentesis is routinely recommended to such women. If signs of Down syndrome are discovered in the cultured fetal cells, the mother is faced with the difficult decision of whether or not to terminate the pregnancy.[3] Fortunately,

---

[1]Medical terms typically owe their origin to Greek or Latin. The word "amniocentesis" is derived from the Greek *amnos*, meaning a membrane, and *kentesis*, signifying a pricking or puncture. The procedure involves the insertion of a needle into the liquid-filled amniotic sac surrounding the developing fetus and withdrawing some of the amniotic fluid.

[2]When amniocentesis first became available, it captured the imaginations of some theologians who opposed the procedure because no informed consent could be obtained from the fetus. The argument is presented forcefully by Paul Ramsey, who proceeds on the assumption that the fetus has a moral status. See P. Ramsey, "Screening: An ethicist's view," *Ethical Issues in Human Genetics*, ed. B. Hilton, D. Callahan, M. Harris, P. Condliffe, B. Berkley (New York: Plenum Press, 1973) 147-67.

[3]It should be clear that no woman subjects herself to an abortion unless she feels she must. Most women who have an abortion do not regard it as "just another" surgical treatment. Abortion remains, at the least, an unpleasant experience. If one takes the absolutist position that abortion is morally indefensible under any circumstance, then prenatal diagnosis aimed at the selective elimination of genetically abnormal fetuses can have no place in medical practice. Certainly those who adhere to the absolutist position will themselves avoid abortion and will continue to condemn those who condone it.

the vast majority of monitored pregnancies are unaffected, and the parents are relieved of the anxiety caused by the threat of a serious disorder in their child.

The human embryo is only one-quarter of an inch long at the end of four weeks of development (Plate III). Yet, there is already an impressive amount of development in the barely discernible embryo. The four-week embryo has the beginnings of eyes, brain, spinal cord, thyroid gland, lungs, liver, kidneys, and intestinal tract. Its primitive heart, which began beating haltingly on the 18th day, is now pumping more confidently. The embryo is enclosed in a protective cover much as if it had enwrapped itself in a highly exaggerated fold of its own skin. This protective cover is known as the amnion, or amniotic sac. This thin, tough sac does not fit the embryo snugly. The space between the amniotic sac and the embryo is filled with a clear, waterlike fluid, the amniotic fluid. The human amniotic fluid is popularly called the "waters" of pregnancy.

Fetal life would be seriously endangered without the cushioning effects of the amniotic fluid, which protects the developing fetus from mechanical shocks as it floats almost weightlessly. The fetus continually recycles the fluid that bathes it, swallowing as much as 500 ml of fluid each day. The fluid in the cavity is replenished by secretions from the upper respiratory tract, particularly the trachea. Commencing at the end of the first trimester, the amniotic fluid accumulates increasing amounts of nonprotein nitrogens (urea, uric acid, and creatinine). This finding is interpreted as indicating the increasing excretion of urine into the amniotic fluid by the fetal kidneys.

The amniotic fluid cells are sloughed off primarily from the fetal skin and amniotic sac; some are derived from the intestinal and urinary tracts of the fetus. Although the amniotic fluid exists from an early stage in pregnancy, the quantities are at first very small and difficult to obtain without appreciable risk to the fetus. At about 10 weeks, the volume of amniotic fluid is only about 30 ml. It is customary for obstetricians to wait until the 14th or 15th week of pregnancy when the volume has increased substantially. At the 14th week, the fluid attains a volume of 175 to 225 ml (six to eight ounces), from which as much as 25 ml can be safely removed.

In the 1950s, amniocentesis was an important obstetrical procedure for the evaluation of pregnancies at risk for Rh disease in the fetus. Amniotic fluid was withdrawn to analyze the bilirubin content of amniotic fluid with the view of determining whether the endangered fetus should be delivered prematurely.[4] These studies on Rh disease yielded an interesting by-product. In addition to obtaining amniotic fluid, the obstetricians discovered that they were also obtaining cells. Tests showed that the cells came from the fetus, not the mother.[5]

Ultrasound diagnosis[6] prior to amniocentesis has been used recently to aid the obstetrician in evaluating gestational age and in localizing the placenta. Gestational age is initially gauged by dating the duration of pregnancy from the first day of the last menstrual period. Such ascertainment based on the menstrual history of the woman is not always accurate. From ultrasound data, the growth curves of the head and thorax of the fetus can be plotted, and the correct gestational age can be established. Additionally, precise localization of the placenta enables the physician to select the most advantageous site for the amniocentesis puncture. Ultrasonic diagnosis is particularly valuable in assessing the possibility of a multiple pregnancy. With rare exceptions, each fetus in a multiple pregnancy has its own amniotic sac. Hence, it is necessary to

---

[4]Rh disease (hemolytic disease of the newborn) is an example of mother-child blood group incompatibility, in which Rh antibodies of the mother enter the fetal circulation through the placenta and destroy the fetal red blood cells. When the fetus' red cells hemolyze (break down), the hemoglobin liberated from the ruptured cells is transformed into a yellow pigment called bilirubin. The liver usually converts the bilirubin into harmless bile, but the amount in the Rh-diseased infant is unmanageable and accumulates in the blood, turning the plasma into an almost yellow-orange liquid. Bilirubin also accumulates in the amniotic fluid, which serves as an index of the severity of Rh disease in the fetus.

[5]One of the first medical scientists to exploit the unexpected discovery that the amniotic fluid cells were of fetal origin was Fritz F. Fuchs, then in Copenhagen and now at Cornell University Medical College. In the late 1950s, Fuchs's examination of amniotic cells enabled him to determine the sex of the baby before birth, an invaluable tool for diagnosing sex-linked genetic diseases such as hemophilia. In recent years, the means of distinguishing normal and hemophilic cultured amniotic cells has become refined and precise. Thus, prenatal diagnosis of hemophilia, found almost exclusively in males, has become a reality. Since hemophilia is treatable, but presently incurable, many thoughtful critics have pondered whether we are socially and morally prepared to cope with therapeutic abortion of a (male) fetus diagnosed unequivocally as hemophilic.

[6]Ultrasound is a form of mechanical, vibrational energy whose frequency lies above the normal audible limit of 20,000 cycles per second. The pregnant uterus forms an excellent area for ultrasonic study. The sonic beam passes virtually intact through the amniotic fluid and sends back strong echoes from fetal and placental tissues. When the urinary bladder is filled, it acts as a water tank that permits the uterus itself to be well outlined.

sample the fluid in each sac. Most reports of the application of the amniocentesis technique indicate no, or minimal, maternal or fetal complications.[7]

Amniocentesis is performed in most medical centers as an outpatient procedure. The surgical preparation of the lower abdomen does not entail shaving, and local anesthesia of the skin is not even necessary. The skin is penetrated by a 20- to 22-gauge spinal needle with stylet. After the needle is inserted, the stylet is removed when the amniotic sac is penetrated. A disposable plastic syringe (20 to 50 ml) is used to aspirate the fluid. The technique is usually successful on the first insertion and is completed within five to ten minutes. Typically, 15 to 25 ml of amniotic fluid are removed. After the procedure is completed, pressure is applied to the site of the puncture for several minutes. The patient can then return to normal activity.

The amniotic fluid is delivered to the laboratory for testing in a sterile, sealed vessel, often in the syringe into which it was aspirated. The supernatant (clear solution) is studied for levels of alpha-fetoprotein. Many structural defects of the nervous system (spina bifida, for example) can be addressed through measurements of alpha-fetoprotein (see chapter 5). The cells in the sedimented material from the amniotic fluid sample are cultured for chromosomal and enzyme analyses. Approximately 24 days are required to complete the chromosomal studies and 35 days for the biochemical assays. Since the culturing of cells takes several weeks, the enzyme analysis is now being performed, where possible, on the uncultured fetal cells of the original sample. Virtually all chromosomal aberrations of the fetus are ascertainable, as well as more than 100 inherited biochemical errors (see chapter 3).

---

[7]The reported frequency of complications with midtrimester amniocentesis is approximately one percent, but the vast majority of these have been minor complications, such as inconsequential amniotic fluid leakage or vaginal spotting. There are no confirmed reports of fetal injury due to the procedure. However, experience with amniocentesis is so recent that it is presently difficult to evaluate any long-term problems, such as possible unforeseen adverse manifestations in the later life of the child. The encouraging report that amniocentesis is a safe procedure when performed in experienced centers was issued in 1971 by the National Institute of Child Health and Development. See NICHD National Registry for Amniocentesis Study Group, "Midtrimester amniocentesis for prenatal diagnosis: Safety and accuracy," *Journal of the American Medical Association* 236 (1976): 1471-76.

The new era of prenatal diagnosis was ushered in by the dramatic finding in 1956 that the correct number of chromosomes in the body cell of a human is 46, not 48 as had long been held as definitive.[8] The chromosomes prepared from a culture of cells can be seen under a high resolution microscope and identified according to their size (Plate IV). The chromosomes occur in pairs, one member of each pair coming from the mother and the other from the father. The members of one pair of chromosomes—the sex chromosomes—may be unevenly matched. In the cells of a male, one of the sex chromosomes (the X) is large; the other one (the Y) is small. In the cells of the female, both of the sex chromosomes are the X chromosome, each of equal size. The chromosomes not associated with sex are referred to autosomes. Thus, the body cells of the human have 44 autosomes (or 22 pairs) and two sex chromosomes. Each autosome pair has a different size and shape from the others. For easy reference, the autosome pairs are numbered 1 to 22 in descending order of length, and are further classified into seven groups, designated by capital letters, A through G. The G members represent the smallest chromosomes in the human complement and also one of the most problematic in terms of congenital disorders.

The first congenital disorder to be traced to an alteration in the human chromosome complement was Down syndrome. In 1959, the young pediatrician Jérôme Legeune demonstrated the existence of an extra chromosome in the cells of infants with Down syndrome. Affected infants do not contain the normal chromosome number of 46, but rather 47. The additional chromosome is a member of the G group, which comprises the two smallest chromosome pairs (Nos. 21 and 22) of the human complement. Affected individuals are said to display trisomy (three rather than two) of chromosome G, or simply, trisomy G (Plate V). Clinically, the condition is often referred to as trisomy 21 since the 21st chromosome is generally involved.

---

[8]In 1923, Theophilus Painter, the late eminent geneticist at the University of Texas, examined microscopic preparations of human testicular tissue and concluded that people have 48 chromosomes. Two years earlier, in 1921, Painter had observed 46 chromosomes in several clear metaphase figures, but he apparently decided that 48 was the more characteristic number. Other investigators of his day supported the value 48, and this number was then viewed as definitive until 1956. Chromosomes are structures that are present in every human cell and are composed of genes that govern the hereditary traits.

An extra chromosome means that numerous genes are represented three times rather than twice. Since a given chromosome carries a variety of genes with different functions, an additional complement of the various genes would be expected to disturb several different bodily processes. This explains what was once considered an inexplicably strange assortment of defects in patients with Down syndrome.

The incidence of Down syndrome is known to increase markedly with the age of the mother, occurring in about one in 1,600 births at maternal age 20, to one in 100 births at age 40. Among women over 45, one in 40 infants may be expected to be afflicted with Down syndrome. Since the likelihood of delivering a child with Down syndrome increases with the advancing age of the woman, it was immediately surmised that the infant's extra chromosome is acquired during the production of the egg. The process of maturation of the egg is complex and subject to error. It does not always proceed normally. Occasional mishaps do occur in the behavior of chromosomes such that a mature egg comes to contain both members of a given pair of chromosomes, instead of the usual one member from a given pair. Such a mishap (technically "nondisjunction") involving the 21st pair of chromosomes would result in an egg cell that possesses two 21st chromosomes instead of the customary one. This egg cell, when fertilized by a normal sperm, would produce a Down infant that is trisomic for the 21st chromosome.[9]

All the eggs that a woman produces during her reproductive life are present from the moment of birth. In fact, her eggs are contained in her

---

[9]The phenomenon of nondisjunction occurs with other chromosomes as well, often with tragic consequences. Since many more genes are carried in the larger chromosomes than in the smaller chromosomes, trisomies involving the large autosomes, such as those of the A and B groups, do not survive to term. Trisomies involving the smaller chromosomes permit increased chances of survival. There are two autosomal trisomies in addition to trisomy G that enable the infant to survive through birth—one of these occurs in the D group of chromosomes (13-15) and the other in the E group (16-18).

Among newborns, about one in 1,500 has a group D chromosome in triplicate; about one in 1,000 is trisomic for the E chromosome (typically 18). Both trisomic conditions, resulting in an abnormal count of 47 chromosomes, are fatal within the first year of life. Common anomalies in trisomy D (typically 13) include cleft palate (often with harelip), sloping forehead with relatively small braincase, defective eye development, and polydactyly (having more than five fingers). Developmental disorders of the heart and kidney contribute to an early death of the infant. Common clinical features of trisomy E infants are recessed chin, malformed ears, spasticity due to a defective nervous system, and peculiarly pliable fingers.

ovaries months before she is born. At birth, the ovaries contain an untold number of cells known as oocytes—immature or prospective egg cells. The egg of a 20-year-old woman matures from an oocyte that has rested for 20 years whereas the egg of a 40-year-old woman has been dormant for 40 years. The maturation of eggs from the oocyte is apparently impaired with advancing age. In other words, there is a progressive decline in the number of eggs that mature perfectly as the woman ages. By the age of 50, the production of functional eggs is typically no longer possible.[10]

For numerous years medical scientists were comfortable in the belief that the eggs of the human female tend to age or become overripe. The aging of eggs was inextricably linked to the phenomenon of nondisjunction. This simplistic view, however, is not without complications. In fact, recent developments have shown that the simple focus on older women and aged eggs is inadequate.

Newer data indicate that the egg is not always at fault, as previously suspected. In as many as 30 percent of the cases of Down syndrome, the origin of the extra chromosome has been traced to the father. The paternal effect appears not to be related to the father's age but is due to factors that are still unknown. The important consideration is that the extra chromosome can arise either in the egg cell or sperm cell. The evidence is clear that the male may be the source of the additional chromosome. In a large sense, the knowledge that either parent can be responsible al-

---

[10]A number of hypotheses have been advanced to explain the higher incidence of nondisjunction in the oocytes of older women. None of these has been substantiated. In 1968, James German, a geneticist at Cornell University, proposed delayed fertilization as the basic cause of nondisjunction. He suggested that the high risk of Down syndrome may be related to the decreasing frequency of coitus in marriages of long duration. Since sexual relations tend to become sporadic, or at least less frequent, after the early years of marriage, the chances are greater in older women that sperm may not be present to fertilize the egg as soon as it is released from the ovary. Thus, German contended that infrequent sexual relations and the consequent danger of delayed fertilization are important factors in the etiology of nondisjunction. English geneticist L. S. Penrose however, was unable to find a correlation between duration of marriage and Down syndrome. See J. German, "Mongolism, delayed fertilization and human sexual behavior," *Nature* 217 (1968): 516-18; L. S. Penrose and J. M. Berg, "Mongolism and duration of marriage," *Nature* 218 (1968): 300; and J. Fabia, "Illegitimacy and Down's syndrome," *Nature* 221 (1969): 1156-58.

lows both parents to share what the mother usually, and undeservedly, feels as guilt.

Since 1960 the mean maternal age for all live births has declined substantially because of the decreasing number of children born to women over 35 years of age. In the United States, the proportion of all births to women 35 and older has steadily decreased from 10 percent in 1960 to four percent in 1980. Stated another way, women younger than 35 are now responsible for 96 percent of all births. Given the lower average age of childbearing women, the expectation has been that the incidence of Down syndrome would also decrease. The anticipated decline has materialized. In 1960, the rate of Down syndrome was 1.3 per 1,000 live births. Now the rate is 1.0 per 1,000 live births—a 24 percent decrease. Concurrent with the decrease has come a change in the proportion of Down infants born to women 35 and older. In 1960, about 43 percent of the births were to women 35 and older. In 1980, only 23 percent of the Down infants were born to these older women. This substantial reduction during the past two decades has occurred not only because of the changing reproductive attitudes and behaviors of couples but also as a consequence of the technologic development of fetal-chromosomal diagnosis.

In about 96 percent of the cases of Down syndrome, the chromosomal complement will show trisomy of the 21st chromosome. Some of these affected infants are "mosaics" in which some, but not all, cells display trisomy 21 (Plate V). The remaining four percent of Down cases are caused by a complex chromosomal aberration known as translocation.[11] Simply stated, this occurs when the extra chromosome becomes attached or fused to another chromosome (for example, No. 21 fusing to No. 14). Microscopically, such a chromosome appears to have an unusually large configuration (Plate V). Its exceptionally large size is comprehensible because it is actually two chromosomes fused together. Thus, a Down child resulting from a translocation event has the 21st chromo-

---

[11]Translocation is but another category of chromosomal aberrations. The different kinds of chromosomal anomalies may be found in standard texts on human genetics. Among those that may be consulted include J. T. Nora and F. C. Fraser, *Medical Genetics: Principles and Practice* (Philadelphia: Lea & Febiger, 1981); A. P. Mange and E. J. Mange, *Genetics: Human Aspects* (Philadelphia: Saunders College, 1980); and F. Vogel and A. G. Mutulsky, *Human Genetics* (New York: Springer-Verlag, 1980).

some represented three times, but the third is practically concealed on another chromosome (usually No. 14). Unlike Down syndrome associated with trisomy, the translocation type runs in families, opening the possibility that more than one child in the family will be affected.

Fear of recurrence of a chromosomal disorder is an important issue in family planning. If a child is born with an abnormal chromosomal complement, the risk of another child having a chromosomal abnormality is not high provided each of the parents has a normal complement. This is the case for Down syndrome caused by trisomy 21. The risk of recurrence of trisomy 21 is of the order of one percent for couples who have already had an affected child. In the relatively rare instances of Down syndrome caused by translocation, the risk of recurrence is much greater. The higher risk is associated with the finding that one parent actually carries the translocation, but in such a state ("balanced translocation") that he or she is normal in appearance. Stated another way, a parent can carry the translocation without showing any symptoms of the disorder because the parent still has the correct amount of genetic material, although some of it is out of place (translocated). The risk to the offspring of the translocation-type Down syndrome is higher when the mother is the carrier and much lower when the father is the carrier. The chance is one in five that the child will be affected if the mother is the carrier. When the father carries the translocation, the chance of having a Down child is only one in twenty. The reason for this unexpected drop in chance is not known.

It is likely that public acceptance of prenatal diagnosis will increase in forthcoming years. There is a reformation of conscience from one generation to another. Each new generation has a sense of values different from the previous generation. As more couples elect to limit family size, a higher premium will be placed on each conception. Women who continue to seek career opportunities will doubtlessly delay childbearing until the latter part of their reproductive years. It is this group of women who are at a relatively increased risk for bearing children with chromosomal abnormalities.[12] They will likely opt to avert the birth of a defec-

---

[12]The increased risk for advanced maternal age has been shown for congenital abnormalities other than trisomy 21 (Down syndrome). A similar increase in relative risk has been demonstrated for both trisomies D and E and several of the nondisjunction types associated with the sex chromosomes (XXX and XXY, for example).

tive child by the management of pregnancies: prenatal diagnosis and the induced abortion of demonstrably affected fetuses.[13]

Induced therapeutic abortion remains a sensitive and controversial issue. Yet, spontaneous abortion that occurs naturally is rarely, if ever, treated as a delicate issue. Most people do not realize that the rate of spontaneous abortion in pregnant women is very high. One in every three conceptuses are aborted involuntarily, so it is not unusual for any woman to have had an abortion—unknowingly or knowingly.

This astonishing statement may be better understood if we explore what happens to 100 eggs produced by women who are reproducing naturally. Under conditions optimal for fertilization, 16 of the 100 will fail to be fertilized. In other words, after exposure to sperm, the probability of fertilization of an egg is 0.84. Of the 84 eggs that are fertilized, 15 will fail to implant (Plate III). Of the 69 embryos implanted at the end of the first week, 27 of these characteristically will find the uterus lining inhospitable. Thus, only 42 eggs of the original 100 are of such viability as to cause the woman to miss her expected menstrual period. Stated another way, by the time pregnancy is recognizable, more than half the embryos have been lost. At eight weeks' gestation when the embryo is now termed a fetus, 65 eggs of the original 100 have failed to survive. Fortunately, the incidence of spontaneous abortion occurring at some point during 8 to 28 weeks' gestation is very low. In summary, one-third of all

---

Medical scientists generally agree that the clear indications for amniocentesis include the following: maternal age over 35 years; previous birth of a trisomic child or other chromosomal abnormality; carrier parent with a balanced chromosomal translocation; raised maternal serum alpha-fetoprotein; previous child with a neural tube defect; previous child with a metabolic disorder than can be diagnosed *in utero*; woman who is carrier for an X-linked recessive disorder (such as Duchenne muscular dystrophy); habitual aborters (three or more spontaneous abortions previously); and multiple congenital anomalies in a previous child.

[13]Presently in the United States, it is estimated that only about 15 percent of women older than 35 who become pregnant undergo prenatal chromosomal diagnosis. In the rural areas, the figure is substantially lower, as expectant mothers in these regions simply do not have access to facilities in which prenatal diagnostic procedures are performed. Surveys have indicated that the public approves and supports the application of amniocentesis in high-risk pregnancies. Nevertheless, in several regions in the nation, many obstetricians have not referred a single patient for amniocentesis. See B. A. Bernhardt and R. M. Bannerman, "Who gets amniocentesis," *Clinical Genetics: Problems in Diagnosis and Counseling*, ed. A. M. Willey, T. P. Carter, S. Kelly, and I. A. Porter (New York: Academic Press, 1982) 107-17.

fertilized eggs manage to develop to term. In mathematical terms, the probability of a live birth is only 0.31, or 31 percent.

What accounts for the high incidence of naturally occurring, or spontaneous, abortions? The vast majority of the spontaneous abortuses have faulty, or abnormal, chromosome complements.[14] Between the 2nd and 7th weeks of pregnancy, 66 of the 100 abortuses have abnormal chromosomes. The most common abnormalities include trisomy 21 (Down syndrome), trisomy 13 (Patau syndrome), trisomy 18 (Edwards syndrome), triploidy, and XO (Turner syndrome).[15] The incidence of chromosomal anomalies falls to 23 among 100 abortuses between 8 to 12 weeks of age. By the end of the second trimester, the frequency of chromosomal abnormalities in spontaneous abortions decreases from more than 80 percent in the early stages of pregnancy to less than five percent. It may be disconcerting to learn that there is a large natural loss of embryos in pregnancy. The important point, however, is the high efficiency with which nature eliminates abnormal embryos during the course of pregnancy. For every 1,000 chromosomal abnormalities that are present in embryos in the womb, only six are expected to survive to the point of a live birth. Thus, 99.4 percent of the chromosomal abnormalities are eliminated naturally through spontaneous abortion.[16] To cite a specific

---

[14]A detailed analysis of the frequency of chromosomal anomalies in abortuses may be found in J. B. Boué and A. Boué, "Chromosome abnormalities and abortion," *The Physiology and Genetics of Reproduction*, ed. F. Fuchs (New York: Plenum Press, 1974) 2:317-39.

[15]An egg can be produced through nondisjunction that has no X chromosome at all. When such an egg is fertilized by an X-bearing sperm, the offspring will be XO, O signifying the absence of a sex chromosome. Women with the XO constitution suffer from Turner syndrome, an anomaly first noticed in 1938 by Dr. Henry B. Turner of the University of Oklahoma School of Medicine. At that time, however, the true cause of the anomaly was unknown. Women with Turner syndrome have rudimentary ovaries, if any at all, and underdeveloped breasts. Anatomically and psychologically female, they are unable to menstruate or ovulate. Instead of normal ovaries, only ridges of whitish tissue occur, a finding that has caused the term *streak gonads* to be applied. In addition, many authors use the term *gonadal dysgenesis* in place of "Turner syndrome." Affected women are also unusually short, have a peculiar webbing of the skin of the neck, and are of subnormal intelligence.

[16]A relatively large number of women with repetitive spontaneous abortions (so-called "habitual aborters") have been found to carry a balanced translocation. Chromosomal aberrations are a significant cause of spontaneous abortion, not hormonal factors or the innumerable other factors promulgated over the years. See J. L. Simpson, "Genes, chromosomes, and reproductive failure," *Fertility and Sterility* 33 (1980): 107-16.

case, 95 percent of conceptuses with Turner syndrome (XO) are spontaneously aborted.

These considerations are worthy of emphasis since the emotional issues associated with elective abortion of a chromosomally abnormal fetus are cast into a somewhat different light when we become cognizant of the efficacy with which nature (natural selection) eliminates chromosomally abnormal conceptuses. Nature has created a great barrier to the perpetuation of chromosomally abnormal offspring. Nature, however, is not perfect. Some chromosomally abnormal fetuses escape nature's screening mechanism and survive to term. Down syndrome represents one of nature's failures; only 80 percent of Down infants are aborted spontaneously. About 20 percent go on to be live-born. The urgent question is whether we should assume the responsibility of ameliorating nature's shortcomings by actively preventing more Down fetuses from reaching term.[17]

---

[17]The trend in the recent past toward reductions in the incidence of Down-syndrome births to women over 35 years of age is expected to reverse in the next two decades as the large cohort of women born during the post-World War II boom moves into the over-35 category. The 35-49 age category is projected to increase from its 1980 level of 19 million to about 30 million by 1995, an increase greater than 50 percent. In the absence of any reduction in Down-syndrome births through prenatal diagnosis, the number of Down-syndrome births is estimated to increase from about 4,300 in 1979 in the United States to about 5,300 in 1990. Only a dramatic increase in prenatal diagnosis–the utilization of amniocentesis by 75 percent of expectant mothers over 35—can offset the projected twentyfold increase in Down-syndrome births resulting from the anticipated larger number of births to women over 35 years of age. See C. A. Huether, "Projection of Down's Syndrome births in the United States 1979-2000, and the potential effects of prenatal diagnosis," *American Journal of Public Health* 73 (1983): 1186-89.

CHAPTER III

TAY-SACHS DISEASE

P eople are generally united on medical measures that genuinely safe-
guard health. In former days, the common illnesses of childhood
took a heavy toll. Today, many infectious diseases such as measles and
small pox have not only been brought under control by social and medical advances but have disappeared in epidemic form. Improvements in
overall hygiene and nutrition, coupled with the widespread use of vac-
cines and antibiotics, have assured that nearly all children are resistant
to the common illnesses of childhood. The large-scale preventive approach has worked well. Common communicable diseases have become
rare and, all told, much suffering has been averted.

A genetically determined disease differs in several respects from an
infectious disease. Most severe genetic disorders remain recalcitrant to
any known form of treatment. The isolation of carriers of infectious
agents does not apply in the case of carriers of deleterious genes. There
is precious little that can be done to prevent most inherited abnormalities
from expressing their crippling effects once the child is delivered. Reliable estimates indicate that one of every eight pediatric hospital beds today is occupied by a child with a condition in which hereditary factors

played a prominent role. The affected newborn cannot be immunized against the genetic ailment.

Do the foregoing considerations mean that the inherited maladies are less amenable to community-oriented control than are the infectious diseases? We may explore this question by examining a mass screening program that was structured on the basis of a clearly identifiable goal: to allow carriers of a deleterious gene to make informed choices regarding reproduction. Specifically, in 1971, a voluntary, community-based adult screening program was initiated among the Jewish population with the objective of detecting carriers of a tragic disorder of infancy known as "Tay-Sachs." The program enabled couples, found to be at risk by screening, to have children free from the severe disease. Within the short span of ten years, the incidence of births of children afflicted with Tay-Sachs disease has been so dramatically reduced that less than a dozen cases are now known in the United States. The mass screening effort to combat, even eradicate, this disease appears to have been successful. But are there shortcomings to the mass screening efforts? Can the same objectives be achieved by individual counseling with the family physician?

Tay-Sachs disease is a recessively inherited condition that is untreatable and fatal.[1] A fatty substance (lipid) accumulates abnormally in the nerve cells of the brain. The storage of massive amounts of lipid deposits in the brain leads to profound motor and mental deterioration. Affected children appear normal and healthy at birth. Within six months, however, motor weaknesses become obvious as the muscles twitch and the infant experiences periodic convulsions. The muscles deteriorate until the infant becomes completely helpless, unable to extend its arms or move its legs. The ability to walk is usually not achieved and, by the age

---

[1]This disorder derives its name from the two scientists who first identified it: Warren Tay, a British ophthalmologist, and Bernard Sachs, an American neurologist. Warren Tay recorded the first known case in 1881. He described one of the telltale features of the disease, the so-called cherry red spot on the retina of the eye. The red spot can be seen as early as the first few days of life. This spot is not in itself abnormal since it represents the normal vasculature of that region of the retina. It is the accumulation of lipid in ganglion cells adjacent to the spot (a "white halo") that is pathologic. In 1887, Bernard Sachs presented the first clinical description of the disease. By 1898, Sachs recognized a familial pattern in the transmission of the disease and characterized the three principal manifestations of the disorder: the arrest of all mental processes, the progressive weakening of muscles terminating in general paralysis, and rapidly developing blindness.

of one year, the child lies still in the crib. Hospitalization typically becomes necessary by the 19th month. The child becomes mentally retarded, progressively blind, and finally paralyzed. At about two years of age, the circumference of the head reaches a size that is approximately 50 percent greater than normal. Increasing feeding difficulties and repeated respiratory infections (bronchopneumonia) become foreboding. The disease takes its lethal toll by the age of three to four years. There are no known survivors and no cure.[2]

A feature of special interest is that 9 out of 10 affected children are of Jewish heritage. The disease is especially common among the Ashkenazi Jews of northeastern European origin, particularly from provinces in Lithuania and Poland. In the United States, Tay-Sachs disease is about 100 times more prevalent among the Ashkenazi Jews than among other Jewish (Sephardi) groups and members of non-Jewish backgrounds. In terms of annual statistics, one can calculate (in the absence of genetic screening) that 50 children will be born with the disorder each year in the United States, of whom 45 will be of Ashkenazi Jewish origin. More than 80 percent of the cases will mark the first appearance of Tay-Sachs disease on either side of the family. Accordingly, to detect the majority of the cases prenatally, it is necessary to identify the high-risk couples before they have children.

Tay-Sachs disease follows the usual pattern of simple Mendelian inheritance. The disorder is traceable to a malfunctioning recessive gene, and is transmitted to an infant only if both parents are carriers of the abnormal recessive gene (Plate VI). Accordingly, a carrier can marry a non-carrier and not produce affected children. The chance that two carrier parents will produce an affected child is 25 percent (one in four) for each pregnancy.[3] Many physicians are familiar with families in which

---

[2]The ability of parents to cope with Tay-Sachs disease is complicated by the dearth of hospital facilities willing to care for the acute needs of the affected child for prolonged periods. Moreover, the hospital costs for the care of such a patient may reach $20,000 to $40,000 per year, the financial burden being assumed by the parents, family funds, insurance companies, and/or some public agency. Thus, the already massive personal tragedy for the family is also accompanied by a social and financial tragedy as well.

[3]Each of us typically inherits two sets of genetic messages for a given trait, one from the mother and one from the father. A Tay-Sachs carrier has a normal gene (dominant) from one parent and a deleterious gene (recessive) from the other. When the recessive Tay-Sachs gene is paired with a normal gene, as is the case with the carrier, the domi-

the first child born to the couple died of Tay-Sachs disease. These parents have often accepted the 25 percent risk of having another affected child, only to be distressed that the second child displayed the disease. Unfortunately, then, in this type of inheritance pattern, the parents cannot be given assurances (in the absence of prenatal diagnosis) that they would not have another child with the same disorder. Such assurances, if ever given solely on probability grounds, would prove to be wrong too often.

The carrier of Tay-Sachs disease has one abnormal (recessive) gene and, fortunately, one normal (dominant) gene that provides protection from the disease (Plate VI). The carrier does have the potential of transmitting the defective gene to the offspring. If the child inherits the recessive gene from both carrier parents, then the child will be afflicted with Tay-Sachs disease. The carriers—often called heterozygotes—are not as rare as might be supposed. The frequency of heterozygote carriers is many times greater—specifically, 150 times greater—than the frequency of affected individuals.[4] The expectation is that one out of every 30 Ashkenazi Jews is a carrier of the gene for Tay-Sachs. Since no Tay-Sachs patient ever reaches reproductive age, affected children always come from two normal (but carrier) parents. About one in 900 Jewish couples are at risk for Tay-Sachs disease in their offspring.

In 1969, Drs. Shintaro Okado and John S. O'Brien, both then at the University of California in San Diego, demonstrated that the massive

---

nant, normal gene masks the expression of the recessive gene. As a result, the carrier does not manifest the disease. When two carrier parents produce offspring, there is one chance in four (25 percent) that their child will be afflicted. There are two chances in four (50 percent) that their child will be, like them, a carrier. Finally, there is one chance in four (25 percent) that their child will be free both of the disease and the carrier status.

[4]The high incidence of Tay-Sachs carriers would seem to be explained most plausibly by some reproductive advantage for the heterozygous carrier. It has been suggested that the Ashkenazi Jews who lived for many generations in the urban ghettos in Poland and the Baltic states have been exposed to different selective pressures than other Jewish groups who have lived in countries around the Mediterranean and Near East. A possible selection pressure may be that the densely populated urban ghettos could have experienced repeated outbreaks of infectious diseases. Interestingly, pulmonary tuberculosis is virtually absent among grandparents of children afflicted with Tay-Sachs disease, although the incidence of Jewish tuberculosis-affected grandparents from eastern Europe is relatively high. The findings suggest that the heterozygous carrier is resistant to pulmonary tuberculosis in regions where this contagious disease is prevalent.

storage of the fatty substance (specifically, a ganglioside[5]) resulted from the absence of any enzyme (identified as hexosaminidase A) that normally cleaves the large fat molecule into smaller innocuous molecules. Thus, the failure of enzyme activity accounts for the persistence and accumulation of fatty material in the brain cells. In a normal person, the enzyme, hexosaminidase A, can be found in a variety of tissues and organs—brain, liver, kidneys, skin, leucocytes, blood (serum), and amniotic fluid cells. In infants with Tay-Sachs disease, the enzyme is missing from all of these tissues. The practical consequence of these laboratory findings became immediately apparent. Since enzyme activity is absent in the cells of the amniotic fluid of fetuses, a reliable method became available to diagnose affected fetuses *in utero*.[6] It was also established that the carrier parents of affected children have lower than normal levels of the enzyme in their cells.[7] Thus, although the malfunctioning defective gene in the carrier does not cause overt disease, it is detectable in cultured cells.

By 1970, all of the ingredients for a successful genetic counseling program were in place. First, the disorder occurs in a defined population—almost restricted to individuals of Ashkenazi Jewish heritage. Second, the detection of a carrier is feasible through a simple, accurate, and inexpensive analysis of blood.[8] Third, the condition can be diagnosed *in*

---

[5]The lipid responsible for Tay-Sachs disease has been characterized and identified as a ganglioside. There are several gangliosides normally present in brain tissue, each of which exists only in small amounts. In a patient with Tay-Sachs disease, the particular ganglioside (GM_2) accumulates in organelles of cells known as lysosomes. Cell functioning is compromised when the lysosomes become engorged with gangliosides. Tay-Sachs disease is also referred to as a lysosomal deficiency disease. See S. Okada and J. S. O'Brien, "Tay-Sachs disease: Generalized absence of a beta-N-acetylhexosaminidase component," *Science* 165 (1969): 698-700.

[6]L. Schneck, C. Valenti, D. Amsterdam, J. Friedland, M. Adachi, and B. W. Volk, "Prenatal diagnosis of Tay-Sachs disease," *Lancet* 1 (1970): 582-83; and J. S. O'Brien, S. Okada, D. L. Fillerup, M. L. Veath, B. Adornato, P. H. Brenner, and J. G. Leroy, "Tay-Sachs disease: Prenatal diagnosis," *Science* 172 (1971): 61-62.

[7]J. S. O'Brien, S. Okada, A. Chen, and D. L. Fillerup, "Tay-Sachs disease. Detection of heterozygotes and homozygotes by serum hexosaminidase assay," *New England Journal of Medicine* 283 (1970): 15-20.

[8]About 96 percent of the carriers of the Tay-Sachs gene are accurately identified using serum (blood) for the assay of hexosaminidase activity. The majority of the remaining four percent of the carriers are detectable by a more accurate assay of the leucocytes

utero at a time when induced abortion can be safely performed. Armed with this arsenal of information, medical scientists moved rapidly to apply the findings to an attack on the disorder itself in the human population.

In early 1970, a pilot screening program was planned in the Jewish communities of Baltimore and suburban Washington, D.C., under the leadership of pediatrician Michael M. Kaback, then at the Johns Hopkins Hospital.[9] Community education was vigorously pursued for 14 months prior to screening by means of informative pamphlets, newspapers, television, meetings at synagogues, and sessions with interested physicians. The first public screening was conducted in May 1971. Since this pilot effort, comparable programs have been initiated in more than 73 major cities in North America, as well as in Europe, Israel, and South Africa. By 1980, more than 125,000 Jewish individuals of childbearing age had volunteered for the carrier (heterozygous) screening tests in the United States and Canada alone. Approximately one in 28 individuals tested has been identified as a carrier. In terms of absolute numbers, 125 at-risk couples—couples in which both members are carriers—have been identified in which there was no previous history of Tay-Sachs disease in their families. For these couples there was an average risk of 25 percent in each pregnancy that a Tay-Sachs child would be conceived.

Parents are generally unaware that they may be at a great risk of having a child with a severe hereditary disorder. A couple may admit to the mathematical possibility of having a defective child, but statements of probability have little reality to most couples. Only when the real danger is convincingly demonstrated does a couple accept the gravity of the situation. Herein lies the value of the information provided by genetic

---

(white blood cells). The possibility that the carrier state would remain unnoticed after both the serum and leucocyte assays has been calculated at less than one in 30,000. False positives—hexosaminidase activity in the carrier range in the serum of genetically normal individuals—occurs in conditions with tissue destruction (such as myocardial infarction, hepatitis, and pancreatis) and during normal pregnancy. To override the false positives, leucocyte assays are specifically recommended.

[9]M. M. Kaback, *Report on the First Conference on Tay-Sachs Disease Screening and Prevention* (New York: Alan R. Liss, 1977); M. M. Kaback, R. S. Zeiger, W. L. Reynolds, and M. Sonneborn, "Approaches to the control and prevention of Tay-Sachs disease," *Progress in Medical Genetics*, ed. A. G. Steinberg and A. E. Bearn (Philadelphia: W. B. Saunders Co., 1974) 10:103-34.

screening. The screening program informs parents whether they carry the abnormal gene for Tay-Sachs disease, so that pregnancies can be monitored. The intrauterine monitoring of the fetus enables a couple, at a predictable risk for the untreatable inherited disorder in their offspring, to decide whether or not to continue a pregnancy. If genetic analyses show the fetus to be unaffected, the pregnancy may continue without further anxiety. If the fetal-cell studies show the fetus to be affected, the couple, once informed, can elect to terminate the pregnancy if they so choose. In essence, through screening, couples are given the necessary information to act responsibly. The underlying assumption is that knowledge and choice are preferable to ignorance and fate.

In past cases, when parents have discovered through screening and subsequent prenatal diagnosis that they have conceived an affected child, they have opted to abort the fetus. The decision is generally not thought of as a choice between life and death for the affected fetus. The choice is between prenatal death and a lingering, painful, postnatal death. At issue is not the saving of the life of an affected child, but the prevention of undeniable suffering.

In the Baltimore-Washington area, organizers of the screening program used multiple channels of communication to educate the Jewish laity about Tay-Sachs disease. The mean age of the participants was 28 years.[10] Most of the men were engaged in professional and managerial work, while their wives were primarily involved with homemaking duties. Forty-five percent had some graduate training. Seventy-five percent were college graduates and only six persons had no college experience. Approximately one-half claimed an annual income of more than $20,000. Essentially, the group consisted of well-educated young people who wanted more children, regularly used birth control, accepted modern indications for abortion, and knew that prenatal diagnosis represented a solution to the problem of Tay-Sachs disease. The participants learned of the screening by word of mouth, newspapers, and/or television. Only rarely did they learn about it from a physician, even though some pregnant women were receiving obstetrical care. Furthermore, the women discussed the issue principally with families and friends rather

[10]B. Childs, L. Gordis, M. M. Kaback, and H. H. Kazazian, Jr., "Tay-Sachs screening: Motives for participating and knowledge of genetics and probability," *American Journal of Human Genetics* 28 (1976): 537-49.

than with physicians or rabbis, despite the medical and moral issues involved.

Private physicians have stood aloof and have been reluctant to promote the large-scale community screening programs. Many have refrained from referring patients for testing. Several studies have shown that the negative attitude of physicians more often reflects inadequate understanding of the genetic problem than hesitancy on moral grounds.[11] The longer the pediatrician and obstetrician have been out of medical school, the less likely they are to believe that detection of genetic disorders is of much moment. Few physicians have much actual experience with genetic problems, few read about them, and many underestimate the incidence of genetic disease. This is also true of the physician's office nurse. These circumstances indicate that a valuable potential advocate of testing (the physician's office) has not been reached effectively by the community-directed educational material.[12]

The propriety of mass screening and intrauterine monitoring has not gone unchallenged. Theologian Paul Ramsey has repeatedly emphasized that the continual practice of abortion of the genetically defective will, in time, pervert our view toward abnormal individuals.[13] He asks the probing question: Will a woman who is encouraged to abort an abnormal child accept the burden of caring for an abnormal one that was not aborted? Dr. Leon Kass, University of Chicago, is also inclined to

---

[11]A study was undertaken in 1974 by a Committee of the National Academy of Sciences to identify the barriers to physicians' screening for genetic disease. The findings indicate that the medical profession is not, as a whole, ready to accept either the importance of genetic disease or the screening for it. The study suggests that readiness could be increased if physicians had a more penetrating knowledge of genetics, a greater appreciation of the incidence of genetic disease, and a more realistic perception of risks. While it is true that many of today's practicing physicians completed their basic professional education more than 20 years ago, at a time when genetics was not part of the curricula of medical schools, it is disconcerting that basic genetic knowledge has not been acquired through continuing medical education. See I. M. Rosenstock, B. Childs, and A. P. Simopoulos, *Genetic Screening, A Study of the Knowledge and Attitudes of Physicians* (Washington, D.C.: National Academy of Sciences, 1975).

[12]E. Beck, S. Blaichman, C. R. Scriver, and C. L. Clow, "Advocacy and Compliance in Genetic Screening," *New England Journal of Medicine* 291 (1974): 1166-70.

[13]P. Ramsey, "Screening: an ethicist's view," *Ethical Issues in Human Genetics*, ed. B. Hilton, D. Callahan, M. Harris, P. Condliffe, and B. Berkley (New York: Plenum Press, 1973) 147-67.

believe that society will come to treat the genetically defective or otherwise "abnormal" in a second class, inferior manner.[14] He laments that the advent of genetic abortion comes at a time when society has finally succeeded in removing much of the stigma and disgrace previously attached to congenital illness.[15]

Critics dwell heavily on the high anxiety levels and stigmatization that attend large-scale screening programs.[16] Participants who learn of their negative test results are intensely relieved. Those who are identified as carriers are unprepared for the disappointing news and usually express shock and anger. Many feel marked, labeled, or "singled out," when they learn that they carry the Tay-Sachs gene. In some communities where individuals under 18 were screened, as in Montreal, the teenagers felt stigmatized by being identified as carriers. It would seem advisable to avoid screening at a time in life when choice of mate is not imminent, and when self-confidence ebbs and flows. The consensus is that carrier-detection programs are best directed to young married couples. In this way, carrier detection neither imposes limitations on mate selection nor on the reproductive aspirations of couples.

In some communities, the detection of heterozygous carriers has actually been discouraged to avoid psychological problems that such identification might create. An advisory committee in the Dayton community recently opted against a mass screening program for Tay-Sachs disease.[17] The Dayton community contains 6,000 Ashkenazi Jews, of whom 1,800 are between 16 and 45 years old. Assuming a four percent carrier rate, there would be 72 heterozygotes for hexosaminidase

----

[14]L. Kass, "Implication of prenatal diagnosis for the human right to life," ibid., 185-99.

[15]Given such concern for therapeutic abortion, the question of a cure for Tay-Sachs disease arises. One avenue of approach is the replacement of deficient enzyme with normal enzyme, thus restoring lipid metabolism to its normal state. A major difficulty is that the protective blood-brain barrier is so effective as to prevent the entry of the introduced enzyme into the brain cells, which are already severely damaged.

[16]See R. F. Murray, Jr., "Problems behind the promise: ethical issues in mass genetic screening," *Biomedical Ethics*, ed. T. A. Mappes and J. S. Zembaty (New York: McGraw-Hill Book Company, 1981) 478-82; N. A. Holtzman, "Genetic screening: for better or worse?" ibid., 482-84.

[17]M. D. Kuhr, "Doubtful benefits of Tay-Sachs screening," *New England Journal of Medicine* 292 (1975): 371.

A deficiency. Given a 70 percent likelihood of marriage, only two couples in this community would be statistically at risk for an affected (homozygous) Tay-Sachs offspring. If these two couples were each to have four offspring, each with a 25 percent risk of Tay-Sachs, then the purpose of screening would be to prevent the birth—or tragedy—of one child born with Tay-Sachs disease. However, to find this one child, 72 people would have to be identified as carriers. The local advisory committee decided that the psychic burden on these 72 heterozygotes was too high a price to pay for the prevention of a single case.

The alternative to mass screening would be individual counseling by the private physician at the time of actual or prospective pregnancy by the couple. Arno G. Motulsky, director of the Center for Inherited Diseases at the University of Washington in Seattle, states emphatically that "an end result similar to that obtained by screening the total population at risk could be obtained if obstetricians tested all pregnant Jewish women and arranged for the testing of husbands only if their wives showed positive tests. More medically oriented schemes of this type have the advantage of arriving at the same results without alarming the whole community."[18] The physician-patient relationship would provide a confidential channel for the communication of results and advice. Stigmatization would certainly be less of a problem. However, for Motulsky's approach to work, the private physician must be prepared to assume a much larger role in screening—a role that he or she has seemed resolutely unwilling or unable to do.

---

[18]A. G. Motulsky, "Brave new world?" *Science* 185 (1974): 653-60.

CHAPTER IV

SICKLE CELL ANEMIA

L ess than 15 years ago, sickle cell anemia was an obscure, unheralded blood disease. It was not, however, a medical oddity to the thousands of black children who suffered from the ravages of the disease. In a provocative article published in 1970, the physician Robert Scott called to the attention of the health professions that sickle cell anemia is more prevalent among blacks than many highly publicized inherited childhood disorders. Childhood diseases such as cystic fibrosis, muscular dystrophy, and phenylketonuria rarely occur in blacks. Scott characterized sickle cell anemia as one of our nation's most ignored major health problems.[1]

Unexpectedly, in early 1971, sickle cell anemia was thrust into the limelight when President Nixon asked that a special effort be made to combat this grim disease. Through a remarkable series of political maneuvers and exploitation by the news media, sickle cell anemia achieved national prominence. Shortly thereafter, President Nixon authorized

---

[1]R. B. Scott, "Sickle-cell anemia—high prevalence and low priority," *New England Journal of Medicine* 282 (1970): 164-65.

federal support for research and treatment of sickle cell anemia in the amount of six million dollars. In the same year, Senator Edward Kennedy initiated hearings on a national sickle cell law that resulted, in May 1972, in a large allocation of 115 million dollars over three years.[2] The mid-1970s witnessed an extensive campaign aimed at alleviating the suffering from the disease and detecting the disorder through screening programs. The disabling disease finally received its share of medical attention, but the attempts at screening have been met with vocal opposition.

Sickle cell anemia remains an incurable disease.[3] The disease distorts the red blood cells, which normally are spherically shaped (Plate VII). In the affected person, the red cells are contorted into rigid crescents ("sickles") that cannot easily negotiate the thin spaces of the capillaries and cause miniature "log jams." The clogging of small blood vessels can occur anywhere in the body, denying vital oxygen to the tissues, and bringing about the painful "crises" that are so characteristic of the disease. Life expectancy is reduced—half the victims succumb before the age of 20 and most do not survive beyond 40. The clinical picture is, however, quite variable, with some patients having only few crises and mild pains for many years, while others become severely disabled or die at an early age.

Sickle cell anemia is not contagious. It results from a defective gene that is more common in Africa than in the United States.[4] An estimated

---

[2]The American way to launch a triumphant attack on any problem, including the conquest of serious disease, is to focus ("zero in") on the problem with inexhaustible funding and unlimited personnel.

[3]Sickle cell anemia was discovered in 1904 by the American cardiologist, James B. Herrick, during a routine office examination of a 20-year-old anemic black West Indian student residing in Chicago. His symptoms were most unusual. The patient had an undernourished appearance, chronic lower leg ulcers and scars from previous bouts, pallor, muscular rheumatism, severe upper abdominal pains, dark urine, and anemia. The aspect that arrested the attention of Herrick was the presence of numerous crescent-shaped red cells (erythrocytes) in blood smears. The patient was kept under observation for six years, during which time he displayed the painful "crises" that we now recognize as typical of the disease. See J. B. Herrick, "Peculiar elongated and sickle-shaped red blood corpuscles in a case of severe anemia," *Archives of Internal Medicine* 6 (1910): 517-21.

[4]Sickle cell anemia is widely distributed in a broad equatorial belt of Africa; as many as 80,000 affected children die per year in Africa alone. The disease is not confined to the African continent, however. It has been found in Sicily and Greece, and in parts of

two million American blacks harbor one defective gene, but fortunately show no or few symptoms and have a normal life expectancy. These blacks are unaffected because they also carry a normal gene that masks the expression of the harmful sickling gene.[5] These carriers are said to have "sickle cell trait." Two carrier parents, each with the sickle cell trait, have the potential of transmitting the harmful sickling gene to their offspring (Plate VI). One in every 500 black children born in the United States inherits a sickling gene from each parent, and the double dose of the sickling gene establishes the crippling anemic condition. Unfortunately, in the 1970s there was massive misinformation concerning the differences between sickle cell anemia, the condition that disables many of its victims, and sickle cell trait, the clinically asymptomatic condition.

When sickle cell anemia became a fashionable issue in the early 1970s, states rushed into law provisions for screening for sickle cell trait. A well-meaning program, it produced serious problems because of an incredible lack of awareness of this disease by the general public, including health professionals. In some jurisdictions, compulsory premarital sickle cell screening laws were added as amendments to venereal disease testing statutes. This had the unwholesome effect of confusing people as to the manner in which sickle cell anemia was transmitted. Virginia, for a short time, required that all prisoners be screened for sickle cell trait. Not only is such a population not likely to be involved in childbearing, but a negative behavioral profile became associated with the disorder. Legislators in Georgia incorrectly thought a person could be vaccinated against this condition. The title of the Georgia law absurdly

---

the Near East. It has been speculated that the sickle cell gene was introduced into Africa from India via the former land bridge between Asia and Africa. See H. Lehmann and M. Cutbush, "Sickle-cell trait in southern India," *British Medical Journal* 1 (1952): 404-405.

[5]It was not until after World War II that the hereditary basis of sickle cell anemia was elucidated. In the late 1940s, James V. Neel, then at the University of Rochester and now at the University of Michigan, postulated that this blood disease is inherited as a simple Mendelian character. The sickle cell anemic patient inherits two defective genes, one from each parent (Plate VI). Individuals with one normal and one defective gene are generally healthy but are heterozygous carriers. The carrier individuals are said to have sickle cell trait. If two carriers produce children, the chances are one in four that a child will have sickle cell anemia, and one in two that the child will be a carrier. See J. V. Neel, "The inheritance of sickle cell anemia," *Science* 110 (1949): 64-66.

read: "Education-Immunization for Sickle Cell Anemia Required for Admission to Public Schools."

The degree of scientific inaccuracy in industry, schools, and the government in the 1970s was appalling. Persons identified as having sickle cell trait experienced difficulty in obtaining health and life insurance or, if they did get life insurance, the premiums were grossly inflated. Many persons identified as carriers were discriminated against in their jobs and even denied jobs. Many children were told that they could not participate in sports because of the sickle cell trait.[6] In schools, some teachers equated this trait with learning disability. Some people confused genes with germs and thought affected persons carried a dangerous germ.[7]

As physicians gained increasing experience with sickle cell patients, a clearer clinical picture of the malady emerged. Anemia, or the reduction in number of red blood cells, results from the shortened life span of the sickled red cells (erythrocytes). Both the liver and spleen are active in removing the irreversibly sickled cells. To compensate for the heightened red cell destruction, the bone marrow increases its production of red blood cells. Occasionally, however, the bone marrow is ineffectual in producing the extraordinary numbers of red blood cells required, and the marrow may actually cease production, at least temporarily. This is known technically as an *aplastic crisis*. Marrow failure is generally considered the most dangerous aspect of sickle cell anemia. The hemoglobin values drop dramatically, perhaps to a fatal level.[8] A rapid transfusion of

---

[6]The child with sickle cell trait should not be excluded from the more vigorous types of physical sports such as football and wrestling. Such vigorous activities, however, are medically inadvisable for sufferers of the disease itself who typically have low levels of strength and endurance and chronic shortness of breath.

[7]Given this kind of ill-founded, but nonetheless real, misunderstanding of sickle cell disease and sickle cell trait, we have finally, during the last decade, come to the realization that any screening program requires better education starting early in life so that everyone clearly understands the nature of the disease. The fault does not reside only with the layperson. Instruction in the clinical aspects of sickle cell anemia in a typical medical curriculum is still limited. Many emerge from medical school with only vague notions that there is a severe inherited disease that affects an appreciable portion of the black population throughout the world.

[8]Hemoglobin, a substance found in the red blood cells, carries oxygen to all parts of the body. The two defective genes in the sickle cell anemic patient continually direct the manufacture of an abnormal hemoglobin molecule. On the other hand, a child who inherits only one sickle cell gene has another gene that makes normal hemoglobin, giving that person approximately a 50-50 mixture of the two types of hemoglobin in the blood.

packed red cells is the only effective form of treatment for an aplastic crisis.

In children under five, sudden severe anemia and shock may result without warning from a massive trapping of red blood cells within the channels of the spleen. The patient develops nausea, marked pallor, jaundice, and abdominal distention. The distended abdomen results from the enlargement of the spleen, which can trap more than one-half of the blood volume. The congestion and engorgement of the spleen with sickled cells can be fatal. As in other types of anemia, the deficit in oxygen flow is compensated by an increased cardiac output. Cardiomegaly (or cardiac enlargement) results from the high cardiac output associated with anemia. Murmurs are almost always present.

Infants and children are especially liable to bacterial infections. In fact, bacterial infections are a major cause of infant mortality in sickle cell patients. Bacterial pneumonia and bacterial meningitis are the most common infections for which patients are hospitalized. Other persistent sites of infections are the urogenital tract and the bones and joints. Growth is delayed and puberty is retarded. Infertility is common and pregnancy, should it occur, holds danger for both mother and child. Sickle cell anemia in pregnant women continues to be one of the leading causes of death in obstetric cases.[9]

When the relatively rigid sickle cells occlude the capillary channels, the interference with circulation causes injury to, or death of, tissue and painful crises. The frequency of crises is variable and unpredictable. Some patients are crisis-prone and have repeated episodes at short intervals—days or weeks—whereas others may not experience a crisis for months or even years. The pain is often excruciating, throbbing in nature, and aggravated by low-grade fever. In children, the pain is often experienced in the abdomen, which is tender to the touch. The clinical picture may simulate acute appendicitis. Congestion of the spleen is also common in children. The spleen is characteristically enlarged in early childhood but atrophies, or diminishes in size, in later life as the organ

---

[9]In one major hospital during a 10-year period, the sickle cell patient constituted only 0.05 percent, or one in 2,000, of the obstetric admissions, yet was responsible for 16 percent of the maternal deaths. See A. T. Fort, J. C. Morrison, L. Berras, L. W. Diggs, and S. A. Fish, "Counseling the patient with sickle cell disease about reproduction: pregnancy outcome does not justify the maternal risk!" *American Journal of Obstetrics and Gynecology* 111 (1971): 324-27.

becomes progressively scarred and ultimately destroyed. Sickle cell anemia does not manifest itself in the first few months of neonatal life. This is due to the protective action of fetal hemoglobin[10] and the very low levels of the disease-causing abnormal hemoglobin during early life. The percentage of fetal hemoglobin at birth is high, but the quantity drops precipitously as the synthesis of the adult form of hemoglobin accelerates.[11] In sickle cell anemic infants, the proportion of abnormal hemoglobin rises to near adult levels by six months of age. After six months of age, the sickling of red blood cells is a constant finding.[12]

Physicians today can provide care for the patient, but there is no cure. In other words, there is still little that can be done for patients in sickle cell crisis beyond treatment of the symptoms. In 1971, Robert Nalbandian, a pathologist in Grand Rapids, Michigan, reported success in de-sickling the distorted blood cells by injecting patients with large amounts of urea.[13] The effect of urea is transient, and the efficacy of urea therapy has been disputed. Anthony Cerami and James Manning at the Rockefeller University in New York have proposed that the agent that relieves sickle cell crisis in the capillaries is not the urea itself but an im-

---

[10]Oxygen is an essential element for fetal life, yet the fetus lives in a uterine environment in which the concentration of oxygen is relatively low. There are several unique physiological properties of the fetus that ensure it a stable supply of oxygen. The hemoglobin molecule of the fetus, appropriately called fetal hemoglobin, has a higher affinity for oxygen than does adult hemoglobin, carrying as much as 30 percent more oxygen at low tensions than can adult hemoglobin.

[11]Several research groups are pursuing some method that would interrupt the normal progression of hemoglobin synthesis, thus stimulating the production of fetal hemoglobin throughout a sickle cell victim's life span as a prophylactic control.

[12]Clinical manifestations are generally first noted between six months and two years of age. A particularly characteristic feature of the early problem between these ages is the so-called "hand-foot" syndrome, a painful swelling of the hands and feet (Plate VII). These attacks result from avascular necrosis of the metacarpals, metatarsals, or phalanges. The joints frequently become necrotic, and such infarcts of the joints mimic acute rheumatism. In adults, leg ulcers or scars of past ulcers are often seen (Plate VII). These ulcerations result from stasis in small blood vessels and generally occur in the ankle region where the circulation is sluggish. Healing is quite slow; the post-healing scar is lightly pigmented.

[13]R. M. Nalbandian, G. Shultz, J. M. Lusher, J. W. Anderson, and R. L. Henry, "Sickle cell crisis terminated by intravenous urea in sugar solution—a preliminary report," *American Journal of Medical Sciences* 261 (1971): 209-334.

purity, cyanate, that is present in small amounts in most urea solutions. The anti-sickling effect of cyanate appears to be more enduring. Nevertheless, it is accurate to state that a suitable anti-sickling agent continues to elude medical scientists. None is appropriate because of the toxic side effects and the high concentrations required to prevent sickling.

The length of hospitalization for sickle cell patients is usually double that of patients in general.[14] Treatment and management include whole blood transfusions, fluid infusions, and drug therapy. The use of drugs is typically extensive, involving anti-infection agents, tranquilizers, cardiac drugs, diuretics, and hypotensives. The patients are characteristically admitted more than once, and a variety of surgical procedures are performed, of which genito-urinary operations (cystoscopy and urethroscopy) are the most commonly undertaken. There is a need for comprehensive insurance to cover hospital costs and physician fees over the entire life span of sickle cell patients. This is usually difficult to provide because of the poor-risk status of the patient. Most patients experience difficulty paying for insurance because the chronicity and incurability of the disease interferes with steady work.

In 1949, the distinguished chemist and Nobel laureate Linus Pauling and his co-workers at the California Institute of Technology made the important discovery that the defective sickling gene alters the configuration of the hemoglobin molecule. Pauling used the then relatively new technique of electrophoresis, which characterizes proteins according to the manner in which they move in an electric field. It was found that the hemoglobin from a normal person had a different electrophoretic mobility than the hemoglobin from a patient with sickle cell anemia. Thus, two different hemoglobin molecules are involved—the normal type (designated hemoglobin A, or Hb A) and the sickle cell anemic variety (Hb S). The red cells of normal people contain no Hb S and the red cells of sickle cell anemia patients have no Hb A. Both types of hemoglobin are present in carrier individuals. Pauling's paper was published in *Science* in 1949 under the title "Sickle cell anemia, a molecular disease." This

---

[14]S. M. Tetrault and R. B. Scott, "Five-year retrospective study of hospitalization and treatment of patients with sickle cell anemia," *Southern Medical Journal* 69 (1976): 1314-16.

was the first human disease that could be characterized as molecular in origin.[15]

Subsequently, Vernon Ingram of the Cavendish Laboratory in Cambridge, England, devised a method for pinpointing the precise nature of the molecular abnormality.[16] His chemical analysis revealed that sickle cell hemoglobin differs only slightly in its chemical composition from normal hemoglobin. The only difference is the substitution of one amino acid, "valine," in the abnormal hemoglobin for another amino acid, "glutamic acid," in the normal hemoglobin molecule. This difference is incredibly minute, but sufficient to sicken the lives of millions of children over centuries of time.[17]

---

[15]L. Pauling, H. A. Itano, S. J. Singer, and I. C. Wells, "Sickle cell anemia, a molecular disease," *Science* 110 (1949): 543-48.

[16]In 1956, the chemist Vernon Ingram, then at the Medical Research Unit in Cambridge, England, and now at the Massachusetts Institute of Technology in Cambridge, Massachusetts, showed how the hemoglobin molecule is altered by the aberrant gene. He pioneered an analytical technique called "peptide fingerprinting." The hemoglobin molecule was fragmented by a proteolytic enzyme (trypsin) into smaller portions called peptides. To separate the peptides, Ingram used a combination of chromatography and paper electrophoresis. The separated peptide fragments ("fingerprints") showed up on the chromatographic paper. The two hemoglobin molecules—normal and sickle cell— were separable into 26 different peptide fingerprints, identical at every location except one. In other words, there was one particular peptide spot in the sickle cell hemoglobin that differed in its position from the corresponding normal peptide. This particular peptide spot differed in only one amino acid from the corresponding normal peptide. In the sickle cell hemoglobin, the glutamic acid that is normally present in the sixth amino acid position of the beta polypeptide chain is replaced by valine. See V. M. Ingram, "A specific chemical difference between the globins of human and sickle cell anaemia haemoglobin," *Nature* 178 (1956): 792-94; and V. M. Ingram, "Gene mutation in human haemoglobin. The chemical difference between normal and sickle cell haemoglobin," *Nature* 180 (1957): 326-28.

[17]Since persons with sickle cell anemia ordinarily do not survive to reproductive age, it might be expected that the abnormal gene would pass rapidly from existence. Each failure of the homozygous anemic person to transmit their genes would result each time in the loss of two aberrant genes from the populations. And yet, the sickle cell gene reaches remarkably high frequencies in the tropical zone of Africa. In several African populations, 20 percent or more of the individuals have the sickle cell trait, and frequencies as high as 40 percent have been reported for some African tribes. The evidence is strong that the sickle cell gene affords some degree of protection for young children against malarial infection. Hence, in areas where malaria is common, children possessing the sickle cell trait will tend to survive more often than those without the trait and are more likely to pass on their genes to the next generation. The heterozygotes are thus

Counseling for patients is a process of imparting information. It should not consist of giving advice.[18] As a general principle, genetic screening is performed on a wholly voluntary basis. Vaccinations against contagious diseases are often made mandatory to protect the public health, but by no stretch of the imagination are genetic diseases contagious. It is also generally acknowledged that screening is appropriate if the disorder being tested is amenable to treatment. Additionally, screening for the carrier status is of value in that it enables couples to be aware of potential risks to their offspring.

We may now ask: What is the rationale for testing for sickle cell anemia and sickle cell trait? It cannot be for diagnosis or treatment of the disease, since most cases of sickle cell anemia are painfully evident in infancy and the only known treatment is amelioration of the swelling and pain. The major value is in the identification of heterozygous carriers, with the view of informing potential parents about possible risks to future children. The screening for the sickle cell trait in young children (as in elementary school programs) or in elderly persons of postreproductive ages, would seem to be of limited benefit. The testing program would achieve the greatest advantage if it were directed toward mature persons contemplating bearing children.

In the last several years, techniques have been devised for the prenatal diagnosis of sickle cell anemia. In one procedure, a sample of blood is obtained by fetoscopy.[19] Only a very small amount of fetal blood from the placenta (0.1 cubic centimeters) is needed to biochemically examine the synthesis of the hemoglobin molecule in the fetal red cells. The tech-

---

superior in fitness to both homozygotes, which are likely to succumb either to anemia on the one hand or malaria on the other hand.

In a similar finding, evidence exists that persons whose red blood cells are deficient in the enzyme G6PD (glucose-6-phosphate-dehydrogenase) are also less likely to be affected by malaria. Data also show a strong correlation between the incidence of malaria and the frequency of thalassemia in the Italian peninsula and in Sardinia. Malaria apparently has had a profound influence on human events.

[18]M. Lappé, J. M. Gustafson, and R. Roblin, "Ethical and social issues in screening for genetic disease," *New England Journal of Medicine* 286 (1972): 1129-32.

[19]The fetoscope contains a small blood-sampling needle attached to a syringe, by which blood is aspirated from the punctured vessels of the placenta. The determination of hemoglobin in fetal blood is accomplished by measuring the uptake of radioactive amino acids in the hemoglobin molecule. The technique of fetoscopy has been used sparingly and has been attempted only by experienced, skilled surgeons.

nique of fetoscopy is not without hazard. Even in the most experienced hands, there is a real chance of harm to the fetus due to infection or separation of the placenta. Fetal deaths with attendant risks to the mother occur in approximately two percent of the cases, or two in 100. Because of the risks and specialized skill that is required, fetoscopy is currently available only at a very few medical centers in the nation. Since 1978, fetal samples for the prenatal diagnosis of sickle cell anemia have been obtained by the much more widely available and safer technique of amniocentesis. The amniotic fetal cells are analyzed for the abnormal sickling gene by methods that take advantage of the recently developed techniques in molecular biology.[20]

There are important ethical questions that accompany these medical advances. Should parents assume the current risks and proceed with the prenatal diagnosis of sickle cell anemia? On what basis should fetoscopy, or amniocentesis, be undertaken? Should a physician admit a pregnant woman to prenatal diagnosis only if the woman intends to abort the fetus if it can be unequivocally demonstrated that the fetus is afflicted with sickle cell anemia? Should the woman be admitted to prenatal diagnosis who has no intention to abort, but who desires only knowledge to prepare more fully in the event of sickle cell anemia in her infant?

Let us assume that the parents elect prenatal diagnosis with the view toward therapeutic abortion, if necessary. Some would argue that abortion is ethically justified as there is no effective therapy for the defect, and the afflicted child would be significantly burdened by the malformation in later life. Some would also contend that abortion is ethically justified when the defect has a predictable course of certain early death. In Tay-Sachs disease, for example, all infants die by three or four years of age and that infant's chance of having a normal life is virtually zero. Sickle cell anemia, however, does not have a predictable course. Parents cannot forecast whether their offspring *in utero*, afflicted with sickle cell

---

[20]The most recent prenatal tests for sickle cell anemia involve analyzing DNA markers near the gene for beta-globin synthesis or examining DNA at the actual mutation site of the gene responsible for the synthesis of the beta chain of the hemoglobin molecule. See Y. W. Kan and A. M. Dozy, "Polymorphism of DNA sequence adjacent to human β globin structural gene: Relationship to sickle mutation," *Proceedings of the National Academy of Sciences* 75 (1978): 5631-35; and R. F. Geever, L. B. Wilson, P. F. Milner, M. Bittner, and J. T. Wilson, "Direct identification of sickle cell anemia by blot hybridization," *Proceedings of the National Academy of Sciences* 78 (1981): 5081-85.

anemia, will be among the unfortunate who suffer excruciating pains and die in infancy, or is among the more fortunate who have relatively minor pains and live fairly normal lives, at least for 30 years. Thus, the information on which the parents must decide ranges from the worst-case scenario to the best-case scenario. Given the unpredictable variability of severity of sickle cell anemia, how do parents decide?

CHAPTER V

SPINA BIFIDA

I n a scene that is far too familiar and remediless, an infant is born with severe hydrocephalus (popularly called "water on the brain") and dies shortly after birth.[1] The parents are assured that there is, at best, only one chance in a hundred that a second child would have the same disability. The assuaged mother becomes pregnant again and, occasionally, her next-born not only has hydrocephalus but also an irreparable form of spina bifida. This scenario need not happen again. Today spina

---

[1]The most important components of the human body are formed very early in the developing embryo. Clearly, indispensable structures are the brain and spinal cord, which appear in rudimentary form before the embryo is scarcely three weeks old (Plate III). A hollow, pipelike tube, known as the neural tube, forms down the middle of the embryo's future back. The anterior part of this tube will expand and thicken to form the brain, while the posterior part gives rise to the spinal cord. The spinal cord is like a cable that transmits messages from the control centers of the brain to various parts of the body through a network of nerves that branch out from the cord. At every level, from the neck to the lower back, the nerves emerge from the spinal cord through openings between ringlike bones called vertebrae. There are 33 supporting vertebrae that link to form the protective backbone. The spinal cord and the brain are bathed in *cerebrospinal fluid*, which in turn is enveloped by membranous coverings known as *meninges*. The fluid and meninges together act as a shock absorber to cushion the delicate brain and spinal cord.

bifida can be diagnosed prenatally in almost all cases, and the gnawing anxiety of the parents can be averted.

Many parents have never heard of spina bifida, and most have no real appreciation of the complications of this congenital disorder. The professional jargon used in explaining this anatomical defect is formidable. Too often, this spinal malformation tends to be minimized when the mother is first told of the disorder of her newborn. Quite frequently, parents gain the impression that an operation would restore the child to completely normal function. Only those parents who have experienced an affected child are keenly cognizant of the attendant serious problems.

Defects of the spinal cord are among the most severe of congenital malformations.[2] In about two infants in every 1,000, the backbone that protects the delicate spinal cord does not form properly. There are 33 ringlike bones—vertebrae—that link to form the backbone. In the normal development of each ringlike vertebra, two lateral plates fuse in the middle to form a single bone that encircles the spinal cord. When the two plates of bone fail to close over the spinal cord, a bony spur is left at each side of the open spinal cord. Since the vertebra appears to be split into two spurs, the abnormal condition is appropriately called *spina bifida* (literally, "two-part spine").

The seriousness of the vertebral defect depends on whether the spinal cord itself and its nerves protrude from the backbone. Fortunately, the most common type of spina bifida does not involve an outgrowth, or herniation, of the spinal cord or nerves. This mild, symptomless type of spina bifida may go undetected or be discovered only by chance on an X ray film taken for some other purpose. There

---

[2] A congenital spinal abnormality is but one of a group of malformations associated with the embryonic neural tube, the future spinal cord. The cluster of abnormalities is referred to collectively as "neural tube defects." These defects range from the fatal malformation known as anencephaly to minor abnormalities in which one or more lumbar vertebrae are mildly distorted. Anencephaly is the virtual absence of the brain—the cerebral hemispheres are completely missing or reduced to small masses attached to the base of the skull. Anencephalic infants are stillborn or die shortly after birth.

In an anencephalic fetus, the centers in the brain that should control the swallowing apparatus are poorly developed. Since the swallowing mechanism is impaired, the amniotic fluid is not properly circulated and often accumulates excessively. This excessive accumulation of amniotic fluid ("polyhydramnios") is a diagnostic sign in detecting anencephaly.

may be a small depression, or dimple, in the skin of the lower back at the site of the defect. When there is no obvious symptom, the condition is called *spina bifida occulta*, the name signifying that the defect is hidden and of little consequence (Plate VIII).

In the more complicated cases of spina bifida, the bluish-white coverings of the spinal cord (meninges) slip through the bony opening to form a cyst-like sac on the baby's back. The hernial protrusion of the meninges is called a *meningocele* and is surgically correctable. In the most severe form of spina bifida, the cyst-like sac contains a displaced portion of the spinal cord itself as well as spinal nerves. This state, referred to as a *myelomeningocele*, is quite serious as the spinal cord is no longer held safely within the backbone. Myelomeningoceles occur five to ten times more often than meningoceles, and although amenable to repair, the prognosis for a normal life is not at all favorable.

There are troublesome complications in patients with myelomeningoceles. The parts of the body under the control of the defective nerves of the protruding spinal cord usually do not function properly. There is typically muscle weakness in the lower trunk and moderate to severe paralysis of the legs. The defect eventuates a loss of awareness of sensations (touch, pain, pressure, and heat or cold) in those areas of the skin normally innervated by nerves. Problems in bladder and bowel innervation usually result in incontinence, the continual leaking of urine and stool.

In the severe forms of spina bifida, the cerebrospinal fluid leaks out and the cyst may be raw and ulcerated. Abnormal amounts of fluid may also collect in the cavities of the brain, resulting in an enlargement of the head, or hydrocephalus. Nearly 75 percent of the infants with myelomeningoceles develop hydrocephalus.[3] Where hydrocephalus threatens to be a complication, surgery is performed to shunt the excess fluid away from the brain.

Some 30 years ago, newborn infants afflicted with myelomeningocele died, if not shortly of inflammation of the meninges (meningitis), then eventually of kidney failure and urinary infections. Today, the chances of survival are vastly greater. Except in cases of severe paralysis, the

---

[3]When the doctor or nurse on a routine visit places a tape measure around the baby's head, hydrocephalus is one of the possibilities that is being checked.

spinal defect can be closed, the urinary tract problems can be controlled by surgery and antibiotics, and some patients can be trained to walk with the help of orthopedic aids. Yet, notwithstanding the striking advances in treatment, many affected children must live with paralyzed legs and no bowel or bladder control. The surgical management of a child born with a myelomeningocele has led to an unprecedented cluster of clinical, emotional, and ethical problems.

Spina bifida occurs infrequently in blacks, Asians, and Ashkenazi Jews. The highest rate is found in white populations, particularly those of Scotch and Irish origins.[4] There are curious variations in the incidence of spina bifida according to geographical locality and seasons of the year. In the United Kingdom, the frequency of this spinal defect falls dramatically as one moves from northern Ireland to the south of England. In the early 1970s, the incidence of neural tube defects in northern Ireland was 8 per 1,000 live births as compared to 2.9 per 1,000 births in southern England. Migrants from Ireland apparently retain their strong predisposition, as the Irish in Boston, Massachusetts, have exceptionally high risks of spina bifida. The statistics also show that the births of infants with spinal defects are most common in the winter months, especially January. Fortunately, in the last decade, for reasons unknown, the United Kingdom, as well as the United States, has witnessed a decline in the prevalence of neural tube defects.[5]

The precise factors that are responsible for spina bifida (and other neural tube defects, such as anencephaly) are still obscure. The most recent findings suggest an interaction of genetic predisposition and environmental influences. Stated another way, an hereditary predisposition that might not otherwise reveal itself could be triggered to produce a spinal malformation by subtle adverse factors in the uterine environment. A variety of environmental triggers have been implicated as causative agents. Uterine infections and deficiencies in placental nutrition have been suggested as two such triggers. One imaginative researcher,

---

[4]The incidence of spina bifida is difficult to establish. The condition varies over time, with epidemics occurring occasionally. Moreover, since the malformation often results in spontaneous abortion or stillbirth, estimates that are based solely on liveborn infants are misleading.

[5]G. C. Windham and L. D. Edmonds, "Current trends in the incidence of neural tube defects," *Pediatrics* 70 (1982): 333-37.

as recently as 1972, speculated that spina bifida is associated with the eating of blighted potatoes by pregnant women. The anticonvulsant drug, sodium valproate, taken by some pregnant women, has been implicated as the causative agent of spina bifida.[6] Heavy alcohol consumption by the mother during early gestation has been suggested as inducing spinal defects in the developing embryo.[7] A popular hypothesis is that nutritional deficiencies of the mother are significant in producing neural tube defects, and that vitamin supplementation during pregnancy can prevent such fetal defects.[8]

There are intriguing indications that spina bifida may result when the egg is fertilized late in the ovulatory cycle. Such eggs are said to be "aged" or "overripe." By experimentally delaying the time of insemination of rabbit eggs, British biologist C. R. Austin established that at least 50 percent of the overripe eggs met early death before they even became implanted in the uterus. In guinea pigs and cattle, aging of eggs is associated with a high incidence of abortions, stillbirths, and congenital malformations. With this kind of experimentation on humans disallowed, geneticists grasp at human activities that simulate a laboratory experiment. Women who practice the rhythm method of birth control unwittingly provide insight into the consequences in humans of overripe eggs.

Consider women who abstain from intercourse on the very fertile days, when ovulation could occur, for example, on days 10 to 17 (Plate III). There is suggestive evidence that sexual activity on the so-called safe 18th day, which typically is heightened following several days of abstinence, may be associated with a higher-than-expected incidence of fertilization of aging, or aged, eggs. In turn, the two birth abnormalities,

---

[6]N. A. Brown, J. Kao, and S. Fabro, "Teratogenic potential of valproic acid," *Lancet* 1 (1980): 660-61.

[7]J. M. Friedman, "Can maternal alcohol ingestion cause neural tube defects?" *Journal of Pediatrics* 101 (1982): 232-33.

[8]R. W. Smithells, S. Sheppard, C. J. Schorah, et al., "Apparent prevention of neural tube defects by periconceptional vitamin supplementation," *Archives of the Diseases of Children* 56 (1981): 911-18; and R. W. Smithells, N. W. Nevin, M. J. Seller, et al., "Further experience of vitamin supplementation for prevention of neural tube defect," *Lancet* 1 (1983): 1027-31.

spina bifida and the companion defect, anencephaly, may be associated with overripe eggs.[9]

According to hospital records in Boston, the newborn of Catholic parents have the highest incidence of both anencephaly and spina bifida—a combined rate of 2.8 per 1,000 births.[10] Two per 1,000 offspring of Protestant parents are afflicted, whereas only 0.7 per 1,000 offspring of Jewish parents are affected with both abnormalities. British scientist Raymond G. Cross has attributed the relatively high incidence of anencephaly and spina bifida among Catholics to the rhythm method. This interpretation is enhanced by the low rate of these birth abnormalities among Orthodox Jews, who observe the rule of Niddah—complete abstinence from intercourse for seven days after menstruation. In Orthodox Jewish marriages, therefore, intercourse commences at, or close to, the expected date of ovulation, the 13th day, when the egg is freshly extruded from the ovary.

The lack of any accepted exogenous etiology focuses attention on genetic factors. There is a slightly higher incidence of spina bifida among siblings, and slight indications of a familial incidence ("runs in the family"). Studies of twins, however, have been very disappointing from a genetic standpoint. It is rare to find both members of identical twins affected by spina bifida. The presence of one malformed and one normal twin would argue against genetical transmission since both twins presumably are subjected to the same environment in the womb. It can be debated, however, whether the uterine environment is actually uniform or precisely the same for both members of a pair of developing identical twins.

Analysis of family histories have excluded a simple Mendelian interpretation for spina bifida. There is no single defective gene; rather, the malformation depends on the interaction of many genes (so-called "polygenes"). Polygenic inheritance is a difficult concept, but may be visu-

---

[9]A close association between anencephaly and spina bifida is seen in comparable statistics on annual incidence and in similar frequencies with which both types of malformation occur. The two related defects, however, have different impacts on the sexes. Females are affected more often than males, the deviation in sex ratio being much more pronounced in anencephaly than in spina bifida.

[10]R. G. Cross, "Anencephalus and spina bifida," *British Medical Journal* 368 (1968): 253.

alized by considering such quantitative characters as height and weight. Height, for example, has all degrees of intermediate conditions between one extreme and the other. The varied heights are controlled by many genes (polygenes), and form a continuous bell-shaped distribution. Those at the extreme of the curve—the exceedingly short and the exceedingly tall—are not generally recognized as having an abnormality! In congenital abnormalities, however, we do recognize that those individuals at the tail of the distribution are *potential* candidates for a major disorder. Thus, with respect to congenital abnormalities governed by polygenes, such as spina bifida, the constellation of genes that predispose an individual to the disorder is situated at the extreme of the bell-shaped distribution curve. Not all individuals at the tail of this curve will develop spina bifida, but all who manifest the defect possess a high proportion of genes at the extreme of the curve.

Genetically speaking, then, the greater the number of risk genes possessed by the parents, the greater the probability that they will have an affected child. It also follows that the larger the number of risk genes in an affected child, the higher the probability that a sibling will be affected. Translated into practical considerations, the more individuals in a family who are affected, the greater the number of predisposing genes segregating in the family. Where two children in a family are already affected, the recurrence risk in subsequent children is greater than in a family where only one previous child has been affected. With respect to spina bifida, the theoretical probability of a second child born to unaffected parents is six percent (about one in 17) when the *first* child is affected. The theoretical probability rises to 14 percent (one in seven) that a third child will be affected if the first two children have the disorder.[11]

Fortunately, spina bifida can be diagnosed in the affected fetus early in pregnancy. The amniotic fluid contains a variety of chemical substances that are derived from the fetus. One of these substances is a protein called alpha-fetoprotein that is produced by the fetal liver. In 1972,

---

[11]In reality, the recurrence rate is related to several factors, prominent among which is the incidence of neural tube defects in a given geographical locality. Thus, in southern England, the risk of recurrence after one affected child is one in 25; after two, one in 10. In northern Ireland, the corresponding risks are one in 11 and one in five, respectively.

medical scientists in Scotland reported[12] that the concentration of alpha-fetoprotein is highly elevated when the fetus has spina bifida (or anencephaly). From the exposed, open defects of the spinal cord or brain, the alpha-fetoprotein "leaks out" directly into the amniotic fluid, thereby raising the concentration of this protein. By measuring the concentration of alpha-fetoprotein in the amniotic fluid, it is possible to diagnose prenatally the open defects of the brain and spinal cord.[13] The optimal time for testing is between the 16th and 18th week of gestation. About 90 percent of the cases can be diagnosed accurately, or at least with confidence. In the other estimated 10 percent of the cases, the ordinarily exposed areas of the brain or spinal cord are sufficiently covered by skin as to prevent the leakage of excess alpha-fetoprotein into the amniotic fluid.

Although this test represents a major medical breakthrough in the prenatal diagnosis of grave disorders of the nervous system, there are instances of false positive results—a high alpha-fetoprotein level is found but the fetus does *not* have a defect of the brain or spinal cord. Present statistics indicate that the chance of a false positive alpha-fetoprotein outcome is about one in 1,000.[14]

When there is a high alpha-fetoprotein level in the amniotic fluid of the fetus, it can be expected that this protein will leak into the mother's

---

[12]D. J. H. Brock and R. G. Sutcliffe, "Alpha-fetoprotein in the antenatal diagnosis of anencephaly and spina bifida," *Lancet* 2 (1972): 197; D. J. H. Brock, A. E. Bolton, and J. M. Monaghan, "Prenatal diagnosis of anencephaly through maternal serum alpha-fetoprotein measurement," *Lancet* 2 (1973): 923.

[13]Alpha-fetoprotein is an alpha-globulin that is synthesized early by the yolk sac and then later by the fetal liver. The synthesis in the liver begins around the 6th week of gestation. The highest concentrations in the amniotic fluid occur at about 13 weeks, after which the quantities level off and then progressively decline. Between the 15th and 22nd week of gestation, the levels of alpha-fetoprotein in the amniotic fluid surrounding a fetus with an open neural tube defect are clearly elevated above the levels normally found in the amniotic fluid. By term, alpha-fetoprotein in the amniotic fluid falls to low, even undetectable, levels.

[14]To minimize the potential for false positive results, the qualitative assessment of acetylcholinesterase in the amniotic fluid has been recommended as the primary diagnostic biochemical parameter. This enzyme is produced primarily, if not exclusively, by cells of the nervous system. Elevated concentrations of acetylcholinesterase would necessarily arise when the nerve terminals in the developing nervous system are exposed by injury. See A. D. Smith, N. J. Wald, H. S. Cuckle, G. M. Stirrat, M. Bobrow, and H. Lagercrantz, "Amniotic fluid acetylcholinesterase as a possible diagnostic test for neural tube defects in early pregnancy," *Lancet* 1 (1979): 685.

blood circulation. Theoretically, it should be possible to diagnose spina bifida in the fetus by testing a sample of the mother's blood between the 14th and 20th week of her pregnancy. Such studies have already been performed with very encouraging results.[15] With the available data showing an accuracy of 90 percent, this testing of maternal serum is invaluable since the vast majority of infants with neural tube defects are born to women with no previous histories of such fetal malformations.

In the absence of prenatal diagnosis, physicians are faced with the immense ethical problem of what to do with the birth of an infant with the severest form of spina bifida, myelomeningocele. Up until 15 years ago, few physicians were enthusiastic about treating children with this debilitating defect. In the early 1970s, pediatrician John Lorber of Children's Hospital in Sheffield, England, became one of the leading exponents of early and comprehensive surgical intervention. In recent years, several surgeons, including Lorber, have assessed the long-term results and have expressed second thoughts about remedial surgery.[16] In spite of the most vigorous surgical procedures, more than half the infants with myelomeningocele die, often after a long succession of operations. The survivors face an untold number of operations. Most survivors have hydrocephalus, are incontinent with kidney ailments, and remain helplessly paralyzed. In essence, a child with severe myelomeningocele, even though surgically treated, remains a child with a severe handicap. John Lorber now advocates that those newborns who are severely handicapped by gross paralysis of the legs or a grossly enlarged head should *not* be given active treatment. The infants should be given normal nursing care, together with medical treatment to avoid pain and discomfort.

Controversy continues to surround the notion that those newborns with severe spinal malformations and hydrocephalus should be left unoperated—to die. A disquieting circumstance is that many unoperated infants do not die quickly, but rather linger for many months or years. The quality of survival of these infants is very poor. The alternatives are equally distasteful: we can treat all children with myelomeningocele even

---

[15]J. N. Macri, R. R. Weiss, N. A. Starkovsky, K. W. Elligers, D. B. Berger, "Maternal serum alpha-fetoprotein and prospective screening," *Lancet* 2 (1975): 719.

[16]J. Lorber, "Results of treatment of myelomeningocele," *Developmental Medicine and Child Neurology* 13 (1971): 279-303; and J. Lorber, "Early results of selective treatment of spina bifida cystica," *British Medical Journal* 27 (1973): 201-204.

though many survivors will be hopelessly incapacitated; or we can withhold surgical treatment and let nature take a lingering, painful course.

Is it permissible to terminate the life of the neonate with a severe myelomeningocele? When the physician decides that a child is unoperable, a decision between life and death is being made. The unoperated infant is being condemned to death—sooner or later. By "letting nature take its course," the physician is asked to overlook the increased pain and suffering of both the child and the parents. If the decision is not to operate, should not the parents accept the responsibility of alleviating pain and suffering by sanctioning the early death of their hapless infant?[17]

The practice of withholding medical treatment from handicapped infants has not escaped the attention of the U.S. Department of Health and Human Services (HHS). This agency issued a notice on 18 May 1982 informing hospitals that they could lose federal financial assistance if "nutritional sustenance or medical or surgical treatment required to correct a life-threatening condition" was withheld from a handicapped infant. The notice was personally endorsed by President Reagan and issued by HHS Secretary Margaret M. Heckler who expressed *her personal belief* that not a single infant should be denied care and treatment. Another notice followed on 7 March 1983, issued once again by Secretary Heckler, directing some 6,400 hospitals to post a sign conspicuously in delivery rooms and nurseries, which pronounced that discriminatory failure to feed and care for handicapped infants in that facility is prohibited by federal law. The notice also included the toll-free number of a new HHS "handicapped infant hot line," that would be open 24 hours a day. Any person with knowledge of any discriminatory failure to feed and care for handicapped infants was encouraged to phone Washington immediately.

Irked by the unwarranted and unreasonable federal intrusion, and rankled by the government's encouragement of hot line calls from people

---

[17]The Lorber standards, or selection criteria, for withholding treatment from infants with paraplegia, hydrocephalus, or major congenital anomalies in association with spina bifida have been largely accepted in Britain. Pediatric surgeons in the United States have tended to adopt a program of operating on all infants to close the spinal lesions and relieve the hydrocephalus because the criteria for determining the potential of the affected infant at birth are not infallible. See C. A. Swinyard, *The Child with Spina Bifida* (Chicago: Spina Bifida Association of America, 1980).

who could remain anonymous, several professional associations, including the prestigious American Academy of Pediatrics, brought suit against HHS and its secretary. On 14 April 1983, the medical profession prevailed in its condemnation of federal intervention when U.S. District Judge Gerhard A. Gesell dismissed the regulations as "arbitrary and capricious," and implied that the regulations amounted to vigilantism. The hot line signs came down quickly throughout the nation within hours of the judge's ruling.[18]

Although Gesell largely confined his legal rulings to procedural issues, his opinion did touch on the sensitive ethical concerns. The judge overturned an insensitive regulation that effectively prevented parents from having any influence on decisions concerning their offspring as to whether or not medical treatment is desirable or warranted. Some of the opinions expressed by Gesell in his brief are worthy of note.

> The Secretary did not appear to give the slightest consideration to the advantages and disadvantages of relying on the wishes of the parents who . . . in many ways are in the best position to evaluate the infant's best interests. . . . None of these sensitive considerations touching so intimately on the quality of the infant's expected life were even tentatively noted. No attempt was made to address the issue of whether termination of painful, intrusive medical treatment might be appropriate where an infant's clear prognosis is death within days or months or to specify the level of appropriate care in such futile cases.

[18]G. J. Annas, "Disconnecting the Baby Doe Hot Line," *Hastings Center Report* 13 (1983): 14-16.

CHAPTER VI

THE PKU EXPERIENCE

Although PKU—phenylketonuria—is a comparatively rare genetic disease, most people are familiar with this disorder. Public awareness reflects the widespread practice of testing newborn infants for PKU, a requirement in most states. The results of screening have been spectacular in terms of salvaging young lives. Progressive mental retardation in the infant can be averted only if PKU is detected shortly after birth and long-term dietary therapy is promptly initiated. Since the early 1950s, many phenylketonuric patients have been spared mental retardation by having received a special diet in early life.[1] Without the therapeutic diet, most affected children would have to spend their lives in institutions.

Phenylketonuria is an ailment that involves a specific amino acid—phenylalanine. Amino acids are derived from the digestion of proteins in various foods and are required by the body for both tissue repair and construction of new tissues. An intake of at least 50 gm of protein per

---

[1] In less than three decades, at least 40 million newborn infants have been screened and some 4,000 PKU patients have been identified before irreversible brain damage occurred.

day meets the amino acid requirements of normal adult tissues. There are eight essential amino acids that cannot be produced by the body and therefore must be obtained from dietary sources. Plants, livestock products, and fish generally contain all of them in substantial quantities. One of these essential amino acids is phenylalanine, the culprit in PKU. Normally, the human body uses a small portion of the phenylalanine for tissue repair and converts the remainder into other harmless chemical compounds. Because the infant with PKU cannot properly break down phenylalanine, the compound accumulates in massive amounts in the body fluids and injures the immature developing brain.

The first case of PKU was identified by the Norwegian physician, Asbjörn Fölling, in 1934.[2] Victims are mentally retarded, usually so severely that they are institutionalized. The majority of untreated PKU patients have IQs below 30; fewer than one percent have IQs above 70. Affected persons frequently have a light complexion (blond hair and blue eyes) because the production of brown-black pigment is impaired. Most affected individuals also have postural peculiarities, convulsive movements, seizures, and an unusual body odor described as musty or barny (Plate IX). Untreated, phenylketonuric individuals have a short life expectancy; fewer than one out of four live beyond 30 years of age.

Phenylketonuria is transmitted by an abnormal recessive gene. An affected infant receives one harmful gene from each parent, both of whom are unaffected heterozygous carriers. With each pregnancy involving heterozygous parents, there is a one-in-four chance that the child will have PKU. The incidence in the United States is currently established at one in every 10,000 to 15,000 live births. The disability occurs most often among northern Europeans and among Americans of Irish and Polish descent. The incidence of PKU is low among American Indians and Ashkenazi Jews. Active screening programs in the southern United States have confirmed that American blacks only rarely have phenylketonuria.[3]

---

[2]A. Fölling, "Über Ausscheidung von Phenylbrenztraubensäure in den Harn als Stoffwechselanomalie in Verbindung mit Imbezillität," *Hoppe Seylers Zeitschrift für Physiologische Chemie* (Berlin) 227 (1934): 169-76.

[3]E. E. Blake, G. W. Rasberry, and E. E. Long, "The results of PKU screening in the Georgia Public Health Laboratories January 1967-June 1968," *Journal of the Medical Association of Georgia* 58 (1969): 117-20.

Shortly after birth, the affected infant has an unusually high concentration of phenylalanine in the blood. In a normal individual, any phenylalanine that is not immediately needed for new tissue construction is converted to a slightly different amino acid, tyrosine, which is involved in several metabolic pathways, including the formation of pigment. In 1937, George Jervis, a New York physician, found that PKU infants are deficient in a liver enzyme (phenylalanine hydroxylase) that converts phenylalanine into tyrosine.[4] Phenylalanine thus accumulates in the blood and tissues, and its metabolites spill into the urine and sweat. The level of this amino acid in the blood of the PKU patient may rise to 25 times the normal concentration. Phenylalanine is excreted in the urine in the form of phenylpyruvic acid, one of the metabolites. An excess amount of another derivative, phenylacetic acid, in sweat accounts for the strange body odor of PKU patients.

It is not the lack of tyrosine that produces the abnormal consequences, but rather the excessive amounts of phenylalanine. Its high levels are damaging to the rapidly developing brain tissues of the infants in early life.[5] Brain damage in the untreated patient develops after birth, not before. Within six months the affected infant, if unattended, shows definite signs of mental retardation. Herein lies the importance of the screening test—it is designed to diagnose PKU in newborn infants during the symptom-free period before irreversible damage has occurred. When the dietary intake of phenylalanine is carefully controlled in early life, mental retardation is typically prevented.

The high levels of phenylpyruvic acid in the urine of PKU patients provided the basis for the first neonatal screening test. Phenylpyruvic acid belongs to a class of compounds called phenylketones (for which the disease is named), which turns a striking green color in the presence of

---

[4]G. A. Jervis, "Phenylpyruvic oligophrenia: Introductory study of 50 cases of mental deficiency associated with excretion of phenylpyruvic acid," *Archives of Neurology and Psychiatry* 38 (1937): 944-63.

[5]Technically speaking, brain damage in an untreated PKU patient results from an abnormal milieu of several chemical substances. Phenylalanine is diverted along a secondary path into phenylpyruvic acid and its metabolites: phenylacetic acid, phenylacetylglutamine, and *ortho*-hydroxyphenylacetic acid. Normally present only in trace amounts, these metabolites occur in such uncommon quantities in the PKU patient as to provide an anomalous chemical environment for the developing brain tissue.

ferric chloride. Accordingly, when a 10 percent aqueous solution of ferric chloride was applied to the wet diaper of a child, the immediate appearance of a bright green color indicated that the child might be affected with phenylketonuria. This test was commonly called the "diaper" test. Enthusiasm, however, dampened as shortcomings of the test became apparent. The diaper test was negative for some infants who had high, harmful levels of phenylalanine. A more serious objection was that the diaper test was not effective until the child was about six weeks old. By that time the child was out of the hospital, away from the doctor's care, and serious brain damage could have already occurred without the parents being aware of it.

In 1961, Dr. Robert Guthrie, Buffalo Children's Hospital, devised a sensitive, reliable blood test to detect abnormal levels of phenylalanine in the infant during the first few days of life. Only a few drops of blood from the infant's heel are required to reveal the presence of excessive amounts of phenylalanine. The ingenious test devised by Guthrie is a highly technical one known as "bacterial inhibition assay."[6] After the initiation of feedings, blood is collected, usually on or about the third day of life as the infant has by then received ample amounts of milk protein.[7] This milk protein will usually trigger the telling buildup of the phenylalanine level if a child is susceptible. Inasmuch as a policy of early discharge is common in many maternity hospitals, some newborn PKU infants may be sent home before they have received sufficient milk protein to provoke an appreciable increase in their phenylalanine level. Statistically, the frequency of cases of PKU that are missed when screening

---

[6]The bacterial inhibition assay depends on the growth of the bacterium called *Bacillus subtilis*. Normally, a particular chemical substance, *beta-2*-thienylalanine, will inhibit the growth of these bacteria on an agar plate. However, certain concentrations of phenylalanine in the blood will override the effects of the inhibitor and allow *Bacillus subtilis* to grow normally. The rate of growth is a measure of the amount of phenylalanine added. A phenylalanine level exceeding 4 milligrams per 100 deciliters (4 mg%) in the infant's blood is grounds for suspecting PKU. In the affected infant, the blood phenylalanine level rises rapidly to more than 20 mg/dl and may reach 80 mg/dl in the absence of dietary treatment. The levels in normal individuals are 1-3 mg/100 dl. See R. Guthrie, "Blood screening for phenylketonuria," *Journal of the American Medical Association* 178 (1961): 863.

[7]American Academy of Pediatrics, Committee on Genetics. "New issues in newborn screening for phenylketonuria and congenital hypothyroidism," *Pediatrics* 60 (1982): 104-106.

occurs on the first day is 16.1 percent; it is only 2.2 percent on the second day, and 0.3 percent on the third day.[8] If the baby is discharged within the first 24 hours of the initiation of milk feeding, a second screening test is strongly recommended at or by two weeks of age.[9] Some states, such as Georgia, routinely request a follow-up check of the infant's blood by four weeks of age.

The treatment of PKU consists of limiting the intake of the offending compound. In 1954, Horst Bickel, a German pediatrician, devised a synthetic diet that is nutritionally well balanced but low in content of phenylalanine.[10] The specifications of the diet are uncompromisingly strict. It is not an easy menu to create because most food items (including milk, meat, fish, cheese, and eggs) contain large quantities of phenylalanine. The restrictive diet must be prescribed on an individual basis to accommodate each child's exact requirements of energy. Continual analyses of blood and urine reveal the infant's tolerance for phenylalanine, and frequent adjustments in the prescribed diet are usually required, particularly during the first six months of life.

One of the chief staples of the restricted diet is a milk substitute called "Lofenalac" that is fortified with fats, carbohydrates, vitamins, and minerals. A bright side of the diet is that a high carbohydrate intake is essential to meet caloric requirements, which means that gumdrops, jellybeans, popsickles, and lollipops are acceptable. There are special problems when the child attends school; teachers and administrators

---

[8]The level of phenylalanine in the blood of the baby depends on such variables as the amount of initial feedings, the dilution of the starting formulas in nurseries, and the maturity of the infant's enzyme system. Thus, it should not be surprising that the minimum period after the intake of milk that reliable phenylalanine levels may be expected in the blood has been claimed variously as 24, 58, and 72 hours. See N. A. Holtzman, E. D. Mellits, and C. Kallman, "Neonatal screening for phenylketonuria II: age dependence of initial phenylalanine in infants with PKU," *Pediatrics* 53 (1974): 353-57; and N. A. Holtzman, A. J. Meek, and E. D. Mellits, "Neonatal screening for phenylketonuria I: Effectiveness," *Journal of the American Medical Association* 229 (1974): 667-70.

[9]U.S. Department of Health, Education, and Welfare, Health Services Administration, Bureau of Community Health Services, "Management of newborn infants with phenylketonuria," DHEW Publication No. (HSA) 79-5211 (1979).

[10]H. Bickel, J. Gerrard, and E. M. Hickmans, "The influence of phenylalanine intake on the chemistry and behavior of a phenylketonuric child," *Acta Paediatrica* (Uppsala) 43 (1954): 64-77.

must take measures to ensure that the PKU child avoid "snack time" milk and high phenylalanine foods at special events such as birthday parties.[11] The diet can be adjusted to accommodate mothers who wish to breast-feed their infants. Breast milk contains immunoglobulins, thyroid hormones, and other components beneficial to the newborn.[12]

The administration of a low phenylalanine diet early in the infant's life is especially important. The earlier the special diet is begun, the more beneficial the effect. The crucial enzyme, phenylalanine hydroxylase, develops after birth, or at least is not normally active before birth. Thus, the phenylketonuric infant at birth has not sustained any damage to the brain. Essentially, then, the cornerstone of successful treatment is to curtail the potentially harmful substrate before it has an opportunity to accumulate in the infant. The mean IQ score at four years of age of early-treated children is 92, which is much higher than in untreated or late-treated PKU patients.[13] One of the most remarkable outcomes since the advent of screening a scant few decades ago is that the admission of PKU children to mental institutions has dramatically diminished.[14]

Because the PKU diet has seen widespread use only since the late 1950s, it is still not known whether the dietary therapy must be continued for a lifetime. Opinions on the feasibility of terminating therapy are very divergent. Some nutrition experts have remarked that the rigid diet can be safely relaxed between four and six years of age. Others have advocated lifelong adherence of some degree. There is presumptive evidence that adverse hyperactive behavior and learning disabilities may occur after discontinuance of the diet.[15]

---

[11]U.S. Department of Health and Human Services, Health Services Administration, Bureau of Community Health Services, "PKU and the schools," DHHS Publication No. (HSA) 80-5233 (1980) (hereafter referred to as DHHS Bulletin).

[12]DHHS Bulletin, "Guide to breast feeding the infant with PKU," DHHS Publication No. (HSA) 79-5110 (1980).

[13]E. S. Kang, N. D. Sollee, and P. S. Gerald, "Results of treatment and termination of the diet in phenylketonuria," *Pediatrics* 46 (1970): 881-90.

[14]G. C. Cunningham, "Phenylketonuria testing—its role in pediatrics and public health," *CRC Critical Reviews in Clinical Laboratory Sciences* 2 (1971): 45-101.

[15]R. Koch, C. G. Azen, E. G. Friedman, and M. L. Williamson, "Preliminary report of the effects of diet discontinuation of PKU," *Journal of Pediatrics* 100 (1982): 870-75.

Today's PKU-treated adult women are socially active, have normal fertility, and have looked forward to having normal children. Unexpectedly, the children of PKU-treated mothers have not been normal—nearly all have been burdened by mental retardation. The dietary therapy that has saved the mother from a mental institution has not protected her offspring. Further, the severely retarded offspring is not responsive to an otherwise beneficial dietary treatment. Medical scientists did not anticipate such a portentous event, which is currently one of the most distressing issues for families in which there is PKU. Affected females have been urged to adhere faithfully to the diet until after their childbearing years.

Before screening became widespread, about one percent of the individuals admitted to institutions for the mentally retarded were PKU children. Although screening has reduced the number of PKU children institutionalized, there are, unfortunately, children born under circumstances where testing is either unavailable or has been discontinued. The annual cost of a single PKU patient in an institution today is about $16,000. The cost to the state for the average confinement of 15 years is about one-quarter of a million dollars.[16] The aggregate cost of dietary therapy of a single PKU infant is not known. Treatment prescribed at a hospital after referral by a physician through a health department is subsidized in many states. Testing, family counseling, the workup to establish the proper diet, and the diet itself (which averages $60 a month) is included in the treatment. The cost of screening is, on the average, one to two dollars per test. It would seem to be both medical and fiscal irresponsibility on the part of state legislators to discontinue PKU screening of the newborn. Nevertheless, at a time of rising demand for health services and of funding shortages, PKU testing expenditures have been taken lightly in some communities. In some instances, PKU screening has been discontinued.[17]

---

[16]In Georgia, there are presently 26 PKU children on dietary therapy at various medical centers in the state. Without the dietary treatment, these children would have to spend the greater part of their lives in mental institutions, which would represent an outlay of at least six million dollars.

[17]As an example of the elimination of PKU screening one can cite the discontinuation by the District of Columbia Health Department. A total of 77,000 newborns were tested in three years and not a single PKU case was detected. The cost to the Health Department for tests in hospitals was $135,000. Since 84 out of 100 live births in the District of

Encouraged by the PKU experience, several states have initiated mandatory screening for other significant enzyme deficiencies, particularly those capable of causing mental retardation. Metabolic disorders that have been incorporated into many screening programs are galactosemia, homocystinuria, maple syrup urine disease, and congenital hypothyroidism.[18] Each of these disorders is responsive, at least moderately, to special diets. Galactosemia is an extraordinary disorder in which the breast-fed infant is "poisoned" by the mother's milk. Affected infants are unable to use a particular kind of sugar, galactose, that is found in milk. The untreated infant suffers from malnutrition, becomes severely retarded mentally, and develops cataracts. Characteristically, the liver becomes grossly enlarged. Unattended, the infant usually dies. The treatment consists simply of excluding galactose from the diet of the infant.[19]

Columbia are non-white, and since the frequency of PKU among non-whites is less than 1:100,000 births, the expectation is one PKU case among non-whites every four years. This is so rare a frequency that the allocation of scarce funds was deemed unwarranted. Because the District had no PKU law, the health department terminated the screening tests without recourse to repealing a law. The District's action prompts the question: Should PKU screening be undertaken only with population groups in which the frequency of PKU is relatively high?

[18]One of the major causes of currently preventable mental retardation is congenital hypothyroidism. The advent of screening in the mid-1970s for this condition of undersecretion of thyroid hormone has led to the recognition that congenital hypothyroidism occurs in one of every 4,000 to 5,000 newborns, or more than twice as frequently as PKU. Newborn screening has now made it possible to begin replacement therapy before signs and symptoms of hypothyroidism are manifested, generally before infants are one month old. As in PKU, the earlier the diagnosis of hypothyroidism and the earlier that therapy is initiated, the greater the opportunity for the child to realize his or her maximum potential.

[19]If the diagnosis of galactosemia is made before the disease is too far advanced, nearly all the symptoms of the disease disappear if galactose is excluded from the diet of the infant. The liver returns to normal size, nausea and vomiting cease, and nutrition utilization and growth improve markedly. Unfortunately, this is not true for the mental damage that has been done. Unless therapy of a galactose-free diet is instituted promptly at birth, there is usually no recovery from the mentally retarded state. The damage to the liver, brain, and eyes occurs in the very first few days of life. Accordingly, if the newborn infant is a member of a high-risk group (for example, the sibling of a child with galactosemia), the diagnosis should be made by testing the blood of the umbilical cord for the presence or absence of the necessary enzyme before any milk is given to the infant. Estimates for the prevalence of galactosemia vary widely—from one in 18,000 to one in 70,000 babies.

The widespread screening of infants has led to the realization that not all patients with elevated levels of phenylalanine have PKU. At one end of the spectrum are individuals who have a limited, but not a pathological, ability to convert phenylalanine to tyrosine.[20] The individuals show lower elevations in levels of phenylalanine and its metabolites in the urine than the usual PKU patients, and have been designated as hyperphenylalanine variants (HPV). HPV infants tolerate dietary phenylalanine, have no mental disability or other clinical problems, and usually do not require dietary treatment.[21] The familiar PKU patient is now qualified as having *classical* PKU. Differentiating the classical PKU patient from the HPV as early as possible is important so as to assure that dietary treatment is applied only when needed so that unnecessary emotional strain to the patient and expense to the family are minimized.

At the other end of the spectrum are individuals with abnormally high levels of phenylalanine, as in classical PKU, but in whom severe mental retardation progressively develops despite the curtailment of dietary phenylalanine. These individuals fail to respond to the dietary therapy because of a genetic defect in a second enzyme of the system— dihydropteridine reductase (DPR). The markedly reduced activity of DPR leads to progressive neurological deterioration and a poor prognosis for survival.[22]

---

[20]J. L. Berman, G. C. Cunningham, R. W. Day, R. Ford, and D. Hsia, "Causes for high phenylalanine with normal tyrosine in newborn screening program," *American Journal of Diseases of Children* 117 (1969): 54-65; M. E. Blaskovics and K. N. F. Shaw, "Hyperphenylalaninemia: Methods for differential diagnosis," *Phenylketonuria and Some Other Inborn Errors of Amino Acid Metabolism*, ed. H. Bickel, F. P. Hudson, and L. I. Woolf (Stuttgart: Georg Thieme Verlag, 1971) 98-102.

[21]Recent studies indicate that phenylalanine hydroxylase is not a single enzyme, but a mixture of three slightly different entities, or isozymes. In the normal individual, all three isozymes are present and functional in the liver. In the classical PKU patient, these enzymes are almost devoid of activity. In the HPV patient, one or more of the phenylalanine hydroxylase isozymes has appreciable activity. Although the total enzyme activity may be significantly less than in the normal individual, it is sufficient to metabolize a substantial proportion of the excess dietary phenylalanine. The levels of phenylalanine and its metabolites in the blood and other body fluids are distinctly less than in the classical PKU patient on the same dietary intake, and thus the HPV patient usually escapes major damage to the brain. See J. A. Barranger, P. J. Geiger, A. Huzino, and S. Bessman, "Isozymes of phenylalanine hydroxylase," *Science* 175 (1972): 903-905.

[22]Patients with DPR deficiency suffer from three simultaneous metabolic blocks:

Perhaps the most difficult problems are those faced by PKU females as they grow to adulthood. Phenylketonuric women are at a high risk of bearing mentally retarded babies. These infants show severe retardation even though the phenylalanine levels in their blood postnatally are normal. Additionally, they often have other serious growth disturbances, such as microcephaly, which is seldom seen in classical PKU. Studies have revealed that the uterine environment of the PKU-treated pregnant woman has a relatively high level of phenylalanine. Accordingly, large amounts of phenylalanine pass through the placenta and adversely affect the developing fetal brain. In this manner, phenylalanine acts as a teratogenic agent—an agent capable of inducing an environmental, rather than a genetical, malformation. Evidently, phenylalanine has proved to be more harmful to the developing fetus in the phenylketonuric woman than did phenylalanine to the woman herself.

A recent survey has shown that 92 percent of the genetically normal children of mothers, who had been treated for classical PKU, were mentally retarded, 73 percent were microcephalic, 40 percent had low birth weight, and 12 percent had congenital disease.[23] Even when the phenylalanine levels were only mildly elevated in the expectant mothers, there was a greater than expected incidence of abnormalities in the offspring. There are claims that a low phenylalanine-restricted diet throughout pregnancy might prevent fetal damage, but this approach is uncertain and difficult to carry out.[24] There are encouraging instances in which a strict diet begun prior to conception has resulted in offspring with rel-

---

they are unable to convert phenylalanine to tyrosine (as in classical PKU); they cannot make DOPA or 5HTP, which are essential precursors of the neuronal hormones dopamine, norepinephrine, epinephrine, and serotonin. Thus, a major problem is the lack of synthesis of important neurotransmitters. See S. Kaufman, N. Holtzman, S. Milstein, I. J. Butler, and A. Krumholz, "Phenylketonuria due to a deficiency of dihydropteridine reductase," *New England Journal of Medicine* 293 (1975): 785-90.

[23]H. L. Levy, G. N. Kaplan, and A. M. Erickson, "Comparison of treated and untreated pregnancies in a mother with phenylketonuria," *Journal of Pediatrics* 100 (1982): 876-80.

[24]J. D. Allan and J. K. Brown, "Maternal phenylketonuria and foetal brain damage: An attempt at prevention by dietary control," *Some Recent Advances in Inborn Errors of Metabolism*, ed. K. S. Holt and V. P. Coffee (Edinburgh: Churchill Livingstone, 1968) 14-38; J. W. Farquhar, "Baby of a phenylketonuric mother: Inference drawn from a single case," *Archives of Disease in Childhood* 49 (1974): 205-208.

atively normal development and growth, at least through the first year of life.[25] Some clinicians are advising that women with classical PKU refrain from bearing children.[26]

Given the unpredictability of low phenylalanine dietary treatment during pregnancy, what should be done? If each PKU woman were to have two mentally retarded offspring, then the prevalence of PKU-associated mental retardation within one generation would approach that of the population prior to the initiation of mass screening and treatment two decades ago. Should phenylketonuric women be urged to use highly effective birth control measures? Should they be counseled to opt for adoption? Should female offspring of phenylketonuric women be counseled to avoid childbirth?

---

[25]After a decade of research and testing, the artifical sweetener, aspartame, produced by G. D. Searle & Co., was approved for marketing by the U.S. Food and Drug Administration. Aspartame is made from two amino acids, aspartic acid and phenylalanine. There is no evidence that aspartame intake substantially raises the level of phenylalanine in the blood.

[26]D. B. Brenton, D. C. Cusworth, P. Garrod, et al., "Maternal phenylketonuria treated by diet before conception," *Maternal Phenylketonuria*, ed. H. Bickel (Frankfurt: Maizenna, 1980) 67-71; and K. B. Nielsen, F. Guttler, J. Wever, et al., "Dietary treatment of a phenylketonuric woman during planned pregnancy," ibid., 87-91.

CHAPTER VII

CYSTIC FIBROSIS

Less than 35 years ago, cystic fibrosis was not even recognized as a distinct medical entity.[1] Shortly thereafter, this disease rapidly developed the unenviable reputation of being the most common genetic disease with a fatal outcome in infancy or early childhood. In the mid-1960s, affected children could not look forward to reaching the age of 10, despite the best efforts of the medical profession. Today, this disorder still remains a burden to children, but a limited life span is no longer foreboding or inevitable. Presently, with increased clinical awareness and aggressive therapeutic measures, more than half the babies born with

---

[1]In 1936, Swiss pediatrician Guido Fanconi identified a disease of the pancreas as being distinct from other known ailments and named it "cystic fibrosis of the pancreas." Almost simultaneously, the pancreatic defect attracted the attention of American pediatricians, Dorothy Andersen in New York, and Kenneth Blackfan and Charles May in Boston. Today, we realize that cystic fibrosis of the pancreas is a misnomer since the disease involves many organs of the body. See D. H. Andersen, "Cystic fibrosis of the pancreas and its relation to celiac disease: A clinical and pathologic study," *American Journal of Diseases of Children* 56 (1938): 344-99; K. D. Blackfan and C. D. May, "Inspissation of secretion, dilatation of the ducts and acini, atrophy and fibrosis of the pancreas in infants," *Journal of Pediatrics* 13 (1938): 627-34.

this disorder can expect to live beyond the age of 21 years. Cystic fibrosis has graduated from the pediatric clinic and has become a disease of adults. There is still, however, no known cure.

Cystic fibrosis is not rare: one child in 1,800 is born with the disorder. This means that approximately 2,000 affected newborns may be expected each year in the United States. Virtually all patients with cystic fibrosis are white; American blacks and Orientals are rarely afflicted.[2] Within a decade it may be possible to screen for adult carriers of cystic fibrosis as well as diagnose affected fetuses *in utero*. If this optimistic forecast were to be realized, it would probably trigger the largest demand for genetic screening and counseling ever experienced in this nation.

Cystic fibrosis represents a malfunctioning of the mucus-secreting glands of the body. Normally, a thin, free-flowing fluid is secreted that lubricates the passageways of the lungs and intestinal tract.[3] In patients with cystic fibrosis, a thick, sticky mucus is produced that blocks the intestinal ducts and obstructs the airways of the lungs. Most victims develop pulmonary disease that is frequently severe and progressive. Almost all affected children have a history of wheezing and coughing. The wheezing occurs as air passes through respiratory tubes that have been narrowed by thick mucus plugs. Coughing is the body's cleansing action to push out the sticky, viscid secretions.

Damage to the lungs may appear weeks, months, or years after birth. Before the introduction of antibiotics, affected children invariably died

---

[2]There are no reports of cystic fibrosis among native African blacks. In the eastern United States, 98 percent of the patients are of white descent and two percent are black. The condition occurs in one in 17,000 American blacks. It has been assumed that the presence of the disease in American blacks reflects interracial crossings. See L. L. Kulcycki, G. H. Guin, and N. Mann, "Cystic fibrosis in negro children," *Clinical Pediatrics* 3 (1964): 692-705.

[3]As the passageways of the lungs become blocked with thick mucus, sacs of semifluid material, or *cysts*, develop. The subsequent scarring of tissues with fibers (*fibrosis*) gives the disease its name. In Europe, the term "mucoviscidosis" is popular and represents an attempt to describe with one word the basic nature of the disorder—a viscid mucus. However, even this term is not entirely appropriate as non-mucus producing glands (the sweat glands) are almost invariably affected.

ILLUSTRATIVE PLATES

DOWN (Trisomy 21) SYNDROME

TYPICAL FACIAL FEATURES

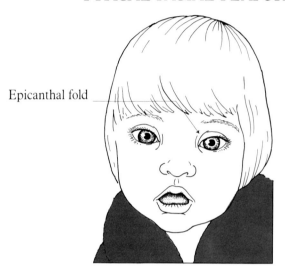

Epicanthal fold

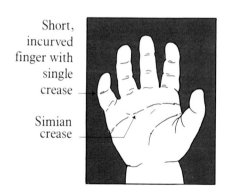

Short, incurved finger with single crease

Simian crease

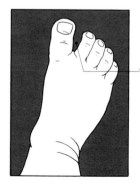

Wide gap between 1st and 2nd toes

Plate I

AMNIOCENTESIS

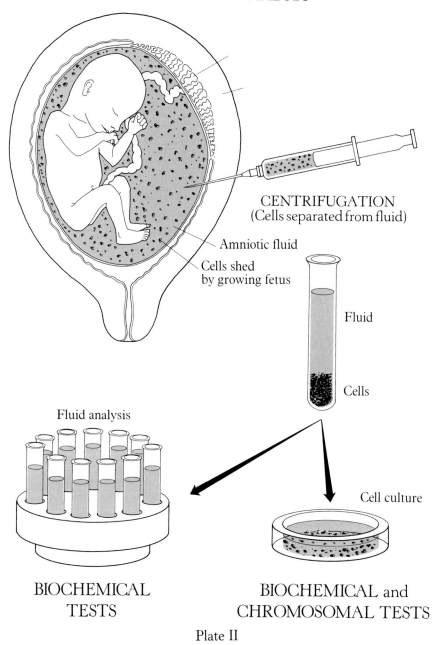

CENTRIFUGATION
(Cells separated from fluid)

Amniotic fluid

Cells shed
by growing fetus

Fluid

Cells

Fluid analysis

Cell culture

BIOCHEMICAL
TESTS

BIOCHEMICAL and
CHROMOSOMAL TESTS

Plate II

STAGES OF DEVELOPMENT

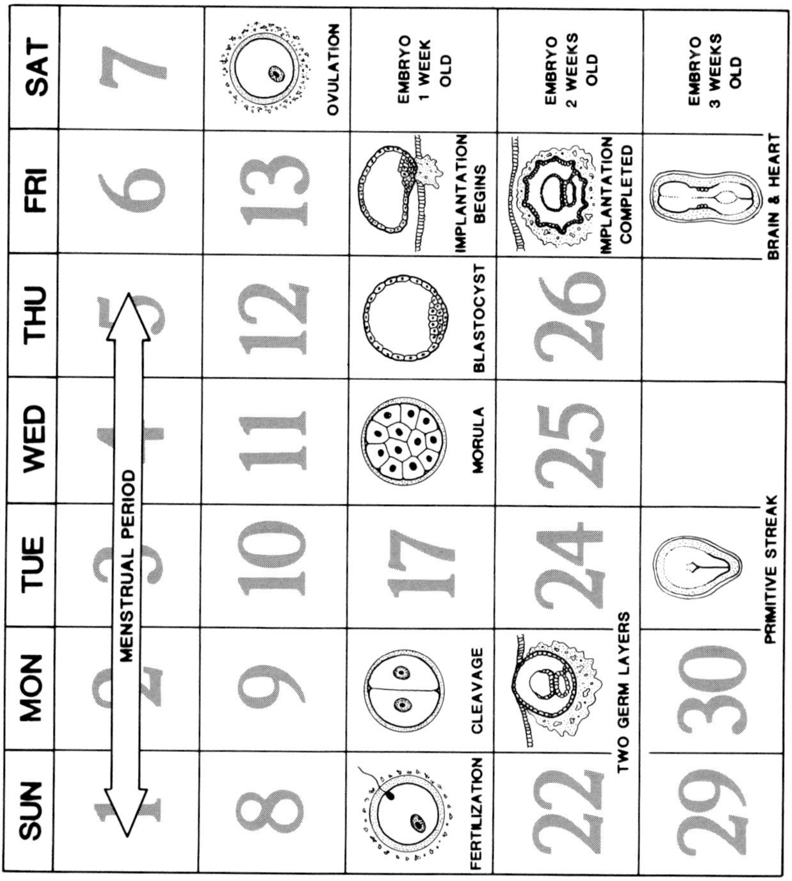

SUN	MON	TUE	WED	THU	FRI	SAT
1	2	3	4	5	6	7
						OVULATION
8	9	10	11	12	13	EMBRYO 1 WEEK OLD
FERTILIZATION	CLEAVAGE	17	MORULA	BLASTOCYST	IMPLANTATION BEGINS	
22	TWO GERM LAYERS	24	25	26	IMPLANTATION COMPLETED	EMBRYO 2 WEEKS OLD
29	30	PRMITIVE STREAK			BRAIN & HEART	EMBRYO 3 WEEKS OLD

MENSTRUAL PERIOD

Plate III

NORMAL CHROMOSOMES
of a HUMAN MALE
(23 pairs, including XY)

CHROMOSOMES
Viewed under
microscope

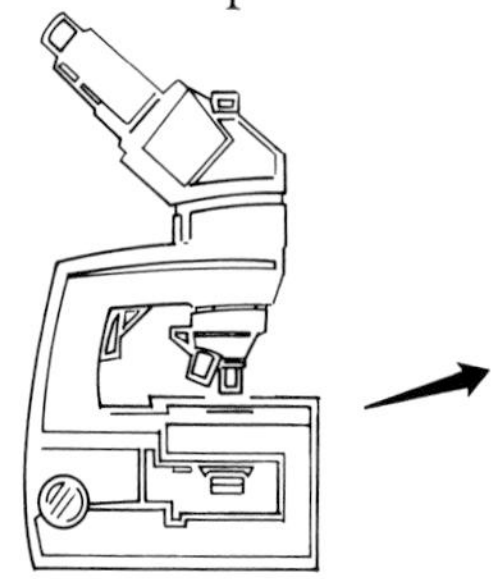

Slide preparation from a
culture of blood cells

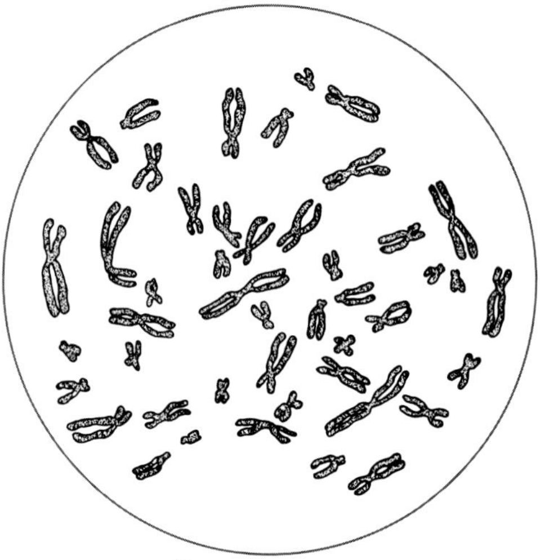

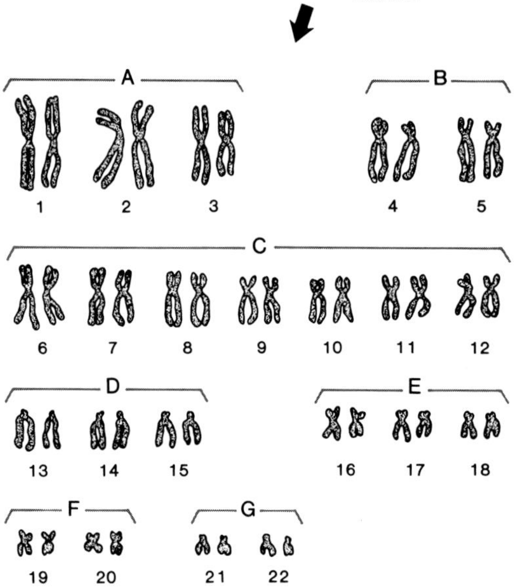

A

1 2 3

B

4 5

C

6 7 8 9 10 11 12

D

13 14 15

E

16 17 18

F

19 20

G

21 22

Arranged in sequence

Plate IV

CHROMOSOMAL ABNORMALITIES
IN DOWN SYNDROME

1. ## TRISOMY 21
    1:600 Births/Rarely Familial

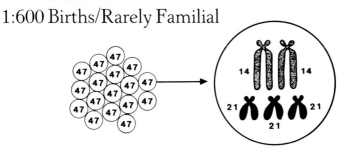

2. ## TRANSLOCATION
    Rare/Familial

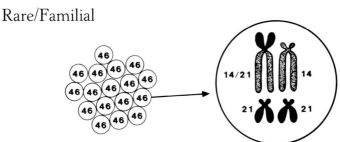

3. ## MOSAIC
    Rare/Not Familial

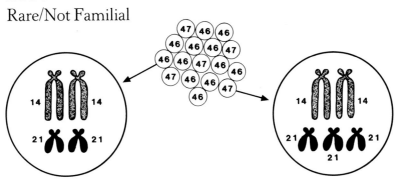

Plate V

RECESSIVE INHERITANCE

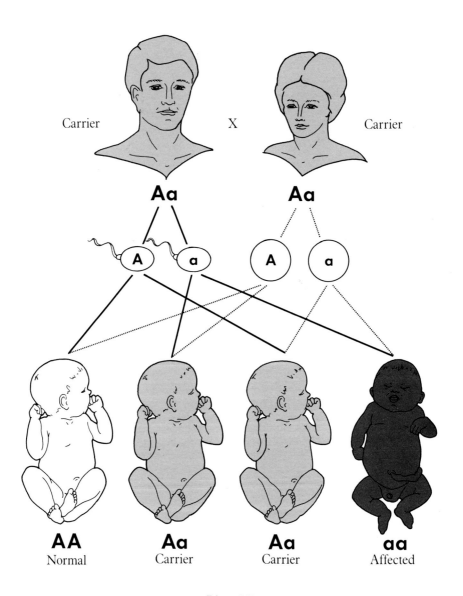

Plate VI

SICKLE CELL ANEMIA

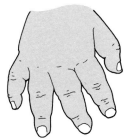

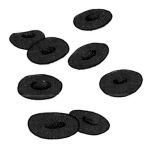
Normal red blood cells

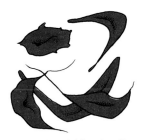
Sickled red blood cells

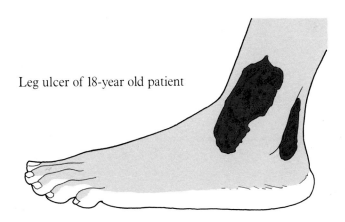
Inflamed fingers of 5-year old patient

Leg ulcer of 18-year old patient

Plate VII

SPINA BIFIDA

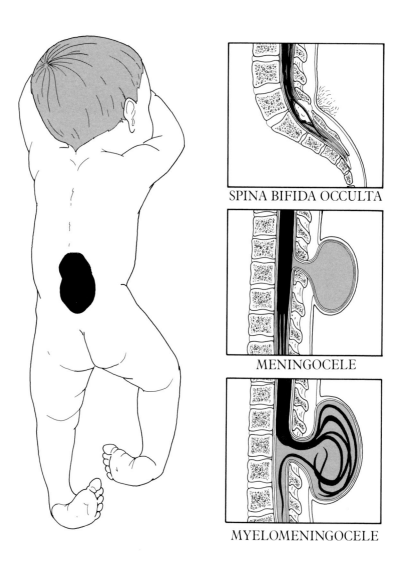

SPINA BIFIDA OCCULTA

MENINGOCELE

MYELOMENINGOCELE

Plate VIII

PHENYLKETONURIA

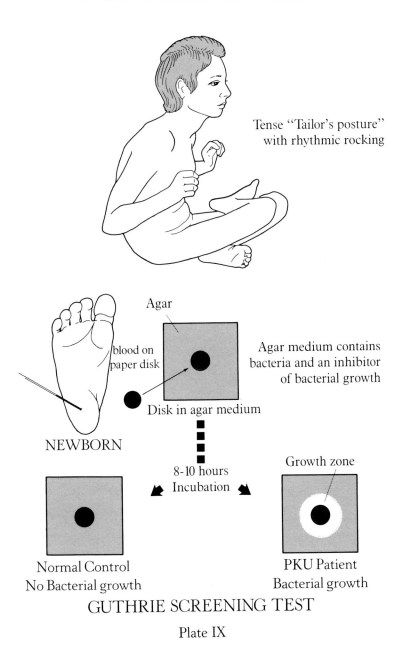

Tense "Tailor's posture"
with rhythmic rocking

Agar

blood on
paper disk

Agar medium contains
bacteria and an inhibitor
of bacterial growth

Disk in agar medium

NEWBORN

8-10 hours
Incubation

Growth zone

Normal Control
No Bacterial growth

PKU Patient
Bacterial growth

GUTHRIE SCREENING TEST

Plate IX

DOMINANT INHERITANCE

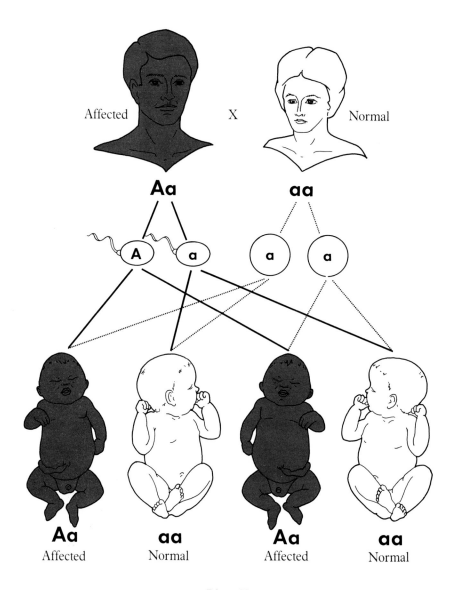

Affected X Normal

Aa   **aa**

A   **a**   **a**   **a**

Aa   **aa**   **Aa**   **aa**
Affected   Normal   Affected   Normal

Plate X

TWO PRENATAL TREATMENTS

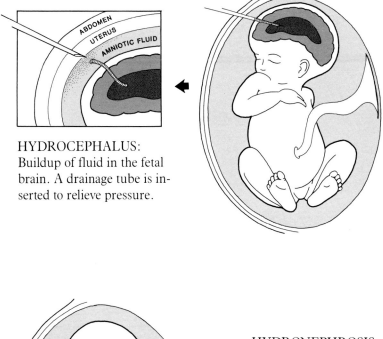

HYDROCEPHALUS:
Buildup of fluid in the fetal brain. A drainage tube is inserted to relieve pressure.

HYDRONEPHROSIS:
A blockage in the urinary tract. A drainage tube is inserted to relieve pressure.

Plate XI

GENETIC ENGINEERING

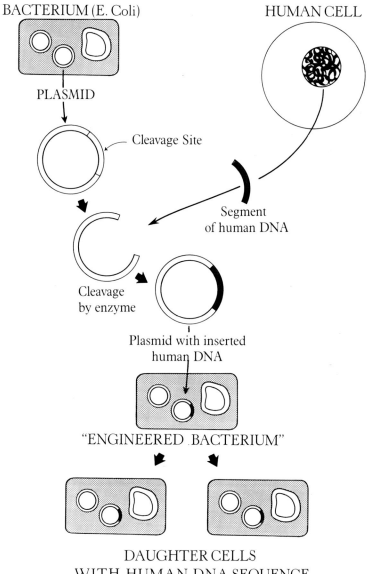

BACTERIUM (E. Coli)

HUMAN CELL

PLASMID

Cleavage Site

Segment
of human DNA

Cleavage
by enzyme

Plasmid with inserted
human DNA

"ENGINEERED BACTERIUM"

DAUGHTER CELLS
WITH HUMAN DNA SEQUENCE

Plate XII

IN VITRO FERTILIZATION

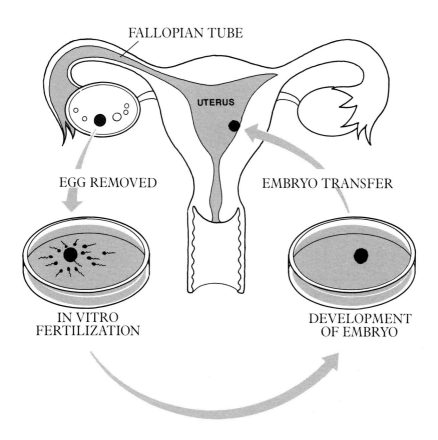

FALLOPIAN TUBE

UTERUS

EGG REMOVED

EMBRYO TRANSFER

IN VITRO
FERTILIZATION

DEVELOPMENT
OF EMBRYO

Plate XIII

in infancy of pulmonary infections.[4] Today, new drugs inhaled as vapor soften the thick mucus of the lungs and enable many children to weather the difficult first years. The outlook is especially bright for patients who are diagnosed before three months of age. The prognosis for survival is dramatically improved with early recognition of the disease, prior to irreversible pulmonary complications. Repeated episodes of pulmonary infections place such a burden on the heart that heart failure may occur. Unfortunately, less than half the diagnoses of cystic fibrosis are made during the first year of life.[5]

Several factors conspire to make early diagnosis difficult. A disease of many disguises, the symptoms of cystic fibrosis vary in expression from patient to patient. It tends to mimic the symptoms of several childhood disorders and may be easily confused with other respiratory and gastrointestinal diseases, such as allergies or gastroenteritis. Only in a very small percentage of cases are the clinical signs of cystic fibrosis confirmable in the newborn. In one in 20 newborn infants with cystic fibrosis, the intestine is blocked by a thick, tenacious mucus material. The classical symptoms of an intestinal obstruction are vomiting and abdominal distension. Surgical removal of this impacted mass of intestinal contents may be required. This obstructive condition ("meconium ileus") rarely occurs in the newborn without cystic fibrosis.[6]

Infants with cystic fibrosis frequently have a large appetite but still appear malnourished. Digestion is impaired by viscid mucus blocking the flow of pancreatic digestive enzymes into the small intestine. Nearly

---

[4]Respiratory complications still cause more than 90 percent of all deaths of patients with cystic fibrosis. Most patients are highly susceptible to lung infections caused by the bacteria *Staphylococcus aureus* and *Pseudomonas aeroginosa*. The latter strain is particularly dangerous and highly pathogenic, since it displays a resistance to most antibiotics currently available. *Pseudomonas* actually stimulates the production of mucin, a major constituent of the thick mucoid substance that blocks the air passages in the lungs.

[5]The delay in diagnosing cystic fibrosis is not limited to months, but may extend to 20 years or more. See W. J. Warwick, "The natural history of cystic fibrosis," *1,000 Years of Cystic Fibrosis Collected Papers*, ed. W. J. Warwick (Minneapolis: University of Minnesota Press, 1981) 13-27.

[6]The dark green mucilaginous material in the intestine of the full-term fetus is called "meconium," and represents a mixture of secretions of varied intestinal glands. Meconium is ordinarily passed by an infant within a few hours after birth. The meconium in the newborn with cystic fibrosis is thick and putty-like, blocking the intestine.

all cases of pancreatic enzyme deficiency in the pediatric age group are attributable to cystic fibrosis. The infant's stools are frequent, bulky, and malodorous. Microscopic analysis of such stools reveals an abnormally large amount of fat globules. This is not unexpected, as fats are poorly digested and absorbed when digestive enzymes released by the pancreas cannot be delivered to the small intestine. Not all children with cystic fibrosis suffer from pancreatic insufficiency; about one out of 10 has moderately normal activity.[7]

Patients with cystic fibrosis are intolerant of heat because of high concentrations of salt (sodium chloride) in their sweat. There is at least twice the normal level of salt. In hot weather, heavy salt loss places the patient at a risk for heat prostration. The inordinately large quantity of salt in the sweat accounts for the "salty" taste of infants when kissed. In fact, the most useful diagnostic test for cystic fibrosis is a quantitative analysis of salt (both sodium and chloride) in sweat. Suspicion of cystic fibrosis is aroused when high values of sodium (over 60 mmol/l) and of chloride (over 60 mmol/l) in the sweat are encountered. However, these findings alone cannot be viewed as definitive, since some patients may have low sodium and chloride levels in the presence of the usual pulmonary gastrointestinal signs. Even normal individuals occasionally show values in the so-called pathological range.

Treatment of cystic fibrosis has been directed at the complications of the disease. The primary focus is on the pulmonary problem. Antibiotics are used extensively to control the low-grade infections that, if untreated, can lead to irreversible, progressive destruction of the lung tissue. Physical therapy is prescribed in the form of a variety of postural positions that help loosen the mucus from the lungs and enable the passageways to remain open. Bronchodilators and decongestants are also useful in loosening the thick secretions. Supplementary salt is usually prescribed to replace the excessive amounts lost in sweat. The great appetite of affected children permits the intake of extra amounts of protein

---

[7]H. Shwachman, R. D. Dooley, F. Guilmette, P. R. Patterson, C. Weil, H. Leubner, "Cystic fibrosis of the pancreas with varying degrees of pancreatic insufficiency," *American Journal of Diseases of Children* 92 (1956): 347-68.

to partially compensate for the loss of proteins in the stools.[8] A low-fat diet favorably affects the character of the stools. To replace the enzymes not released by the pancreas, the child is administered pancreatic enzymes orally before each meal.[9] Although pancreatic insufficiency may be controlled by administration of pancreatic extracts, large and often increasing amounts of the extracts must be given as the disease progresses.

Sexual function is not impaired in the male with cystic fibrosis, but 95 percent are sterile. Almost universally, the sperm ducts atrophy, or degenerate, as a consequence of prolonged blockage by the thick mucus secretions. The female patient does not have a comparable anatomical abnormality. However, her fertility is below normal, as the thick desiccated cervical mucus tends to be inhospitable to the sperm cells. One in every three affected females is married, and among affected women who become pregnant, there is an increased incidence of prematurity and perinatal deaths.[10]

Cystic fibrosis is both an enigma and a challenge to medical science. This incurable disease, sooner or later, is seriously handicapping. The disease has a simple pattern of recessive Mendelian inheritance; the one-in-four risk of recurrence in a sibling is well established (Plate VI). Although one in 20 American whites is a carrier of cystic fibrosis, there is, as yet, no satisfactory test for the heterozygous carrier. In the search for a test for carriers, the presumption is that the flaw in gene activity results in the production of a specific abnormal protein. Investigators have looked diligently for such a detrimental protein, but with only limited

---

[8]Parents often provide useful diagnostic hints to the pediatrician that their child has cystic fibrosis. Parents report that the child eats voraciously, yet fails to gain weight. They remark that the child's skin tastes salty when kissed. They express concern over a persistent asthmatic-like wheezing cough. All these characteristics, indicative of cystic fibrosis, alert the physician to the disorder.

[9]Several tests of pancreatic insufficiency are performed before a diagnosis of cystic fibrosis is confirmed. Such tests include the determination of chymotrypsin activity in the feces, measurements of the content of fat in the feces, evaluation of vitamin levels in the serum, and assays of various pancreatic enzymes, the levels of which reflect the extent of impairment of the pancreas.

[10]L. F. Cohen, P. A. di Sant'Agnese, and J. Friedlander, "Cystic fibrosis and pregnancy," *Lancet* 2 (1980): 842-44.

success. In 1967, pediatrician Alexander Spock and his colleagues at Duke University discovered that a heat-labile protein in the blood of patients with cystic fibrosis adversely affects the movement of cilia.[11] Specifically, when the blood samples are placed on explants of cells lining the windpipe (trachea) of a rabbit, the thin, hairlike cilia that cover the tracheal cells lose their normal, coordinated, wavelike motion and begin to beat erratically. It was then observed that the irregularity of ciliary movement also occurred when blood samples from heterozygous carriers were used. Subsequently, it was discovered that the assay could employ cilia from the gills of the common American oyster.[12] Enthusiasm dampened when it was found that the disorganization of ciliary movement could result from disorders other than cystic fibrosis (allergies, for example). Some years ago, Gregory B. Wilson, Medical University of South Carolina in Charleston, identified a protein by high-resolution biochemical techniques that apparently are unique to patients with cystic fibrosis as well as heterozygous carriers.[13] The existence of this "cystic fibrosis protein" (CFP) has been the subject of appreciable controversy.

The techniques for screening the newborn are presently inaccurate, unreliable, and controversial. No single screening method can be accepted as a final diagnostic procedure. Even the expected increased levels of salt in the sweat of the affected newborn may not be encountered, if only for the cogent reason that newborns actually perspire very little. It is exceedingly difficult to obtain a reliable sweat test during the first six weeks of an infant's life.[14] If the most important aspect in promoting

---

[11]A. Spock, H. M. C. Heich, H. Cress, and W. S. Logan, "Abnormal serum factor in patients with cystic fibrosis of the pancreas," *Pediatric Research* 1 (1967): 173-77.

[12]B. H. Bowman, L. H. Lockhart, M. C. McCombs, "Oyster ciliary inhibition by cystic fibrosis factor," *Science* 164 (1969): 325-26.

[13]G. B. Wilson, H. H. Fudenberg, T. L. Jahn, "Studies on cystic fibrosis using iso-electric focusing. I. An assay for detection of cystic fibrosis homozygotes and heterozygote carriers from serum," *Pediatric Research* 9 (1975): 635-40.

[14]The diagnosis of cystic fibrosis by a sweat test is occasionally erroneous because several clinical conditions may elevate the electrolytes in sweat, particularly untreated adrenal insufficiency, renal diabetes insipidus, and ectodermal dysplasia. To minimize the number of false positive results, experienced laboratories rely on the quantitative pilocarpine iontophoretic sweat test described by Gibson and Cooke. The test results should be interpreted by a physician knowledgeable in the clinical aspects of cystic fibrosis. Sus-

a longer, healthier life is an early diagnosis, then an evaluative test that permits early diagnosis becomes absolutely necessary.

There must be a simple, reliable, and inexpensive method that can be routinely used in nurseries for the purpose of early diagnosis so as to initiate proper therapy at the earliest possible time. Several tests have been proposed, including sweat tests for sodium chloride, analysis of sodium and potassium in fingernail and toenail clippings, and strip tests for albumin in meconium. None of these tests are sufficiently sensitive.[15] The strip test for albumin in meconium, for example, will not detect cystic fibrosis in an affected infant with a functional pancreas. One of the more promising tests with low rates of false positive results is the assay of trypsin in the blood of infants.[16] Because the pancreatic ducts are blocked, trypsin leaks into the blood and is present in elevated quantities in affected infants. The higher concentrations of trypsin can be detected in dried blood spot samples collected routinely for other neonatal screening tests, particularly PKU. Various studies have indicated that the test is diagnostic for cystic fibrosis even when the affected infant has reasonably adequate pancreatic function.

If a reliable method of screening on a massive scale does become available, then a great burden is placed on families and on society to provide adequate resources so that afflicted children can receive complete long-term therapy. At present the families shoulder almost the entire load. As is true in all chronic illnesses, a child with cystic fibrosis often prompts a series of crises in the family. For the affected child, the difficulties and discomforts of living on a daily basis with the disease are often overwhelming. The emotional, social, and financial burden on

---

picion of cystic fibrosis is aroused when high values of sodium (over 60 mmol/l) and of chloride (over 60 mmol/l) are encountered in duplicate trials. Such high values are diagnostic for cystic fibrosis when accompanied by one or more of the following conditions: chronic pulmonary disease, pancreatic insufficiency, or family history of cystic fibrosis.

[15]D. A. Howell, "Report of the committee for a study for evaluation of testing for cystic fibrosis," *Pediatrics* 88 (1976): 711-50.

[16]J. R. Crossley, P. A. Smith, B. W. Edgar, P. D. Gluckman, R. B. Elliot, "Neonatal screening for cystic fibrosis, using immunoreactive trypsin assay in dried blood spot," *Clinica Chimica Acta* 113 (1981): 111-21; B. Wilcken, A. R. D. Brown, R. Urwin, and D. A. Brown, "Cystic fibrosis screening by dried blood spot trypsin assay: Results in 75,000 newborn infants," *Journal of Pediatrics* 102 (1983): 383-87.

families can be enormous. The cost of drugs, diet supplements, and equipment often exceeds $10,000 annually, year after year. Hospitalizations are likely to further increase the financial strain. The need for constant supervision in the daily home therapy programs can bring despair. Healthy siblings have a difficult time coping with the seemingly excessive attention given to the affected child by the parents. Marital relationships are often strained. It is difficult to inform parents that their son, in the unlikely event that he will survive to reproductive age, will probably be sterile.

For many years, numerous attempts have been made to develop a test for the prenatal detection of cystic fibrosis, utilizing either cell-free amniotic fluid or cultivated amniotic fluid cells.[17] The results have been disappointing. However, the thrust for prenatal screening may well be a two-edged sword. The survival of patients with cystic fibrosis has improved dramatically in the last two decades. Nevertheless, the disorder still retains its distressing aspects, and the greater longevity may be viewed as imposing greater, rather than lesser, burdens on the patients and their families. Given these circumstances, what will be the attitude of parents if prenatal diagnosis becomes a reality and a cure has yet to be found? Some parents will opt to terminate the pregnancy. Others will use the information to prepare themselves for the birth and protracted care of a very sick offspring.

---

[17]Studies by Henry L. Nadler at Wayne State University School of Medicine indicate the potential value of monitoring pregnancies for cystic fibrosis by measuring certain proteases or their precursors in the cell-free amniotic fluid. The assay is not consistently reproducible; several unexplained misdiagnoses (false negatives) have occurred. See H. L. Nadler and M. M. J. Walsh, "Intrauterine detection of cystic fibrosis," *Pediatrics* 66 (1980): 690-92.

CHAPTER VIII

HUNTINGTON'S DISEASE

H untington's disease is an inherited disorder characterized by uncontrollable swaying movements of the body and the progressive
loss of mental function.[1] People with the disease were once said to have
"chorea," from the Latin *choreic* for dance, alluding to the strange dance-
like motions of the patients.[2] In the United States, Huntington's disease
is most prevalent in the New England area, where it can be traced back
to colonists in Massachusetts who, in 1631, left England in the famous

---

[1]A clear and comprehensive clinical description of the disease was first presented in
1872 by American physician George S. Huntington, based on his experience with choreic patients on Long Island in New York (*Medical and Surgical Reporter* 26 [1872]: 317-
21). The paper, "On chorea," was Huntington's only manuscript to appear in print. In
tribute to his analysis, in which he accurately discerned the hereditary transmissability,
the disorder was named "Huntington's chorea." Since there are aspects to the disease
other than disorganized muscular movements, the more general term, "Huntington's
disease," is preferred today.

[2]In Germany during the Middle Ages, the disease of "dancing mania" was called *St.
Johannes chorea*, after St. John the Baptist, the patron saint who guarded against disorganized body movement. Later, the "dancing plague" or "twitches" was christened
Chorea St. Vitus dance, when St. Vitus became the patron saint of all afflicted with in-
cessant, jerky movements.

fleet organized by the puritanical anti-Royalist John Winthrop. Of these early colonists only three or four families are held to be responsible for transmitting the disorder to all subsequent generations. Today, it is estimated that there may be as many as 25,000 persons in the United States afflicted with the disorder. Huntington's disease was then termed *magrums*, meaning "fidgets" or "mad staggers." The involuntary jerking and twisting of the arms and legs was considered a curse inherited by the choreics from their forefathers for having blasphemously imitated Christ during crucifixion. In colonial New England, from 1646 to 1697, choreic women were denounced as witches and were persecuted.

The symptoms usually develop in an affected person between the ages of 30 and 45.[3] There is no cure and the progress of the disease is relentless, leading to a terminal state of helplessness. There is no therapy that can significantly alter the natural progression of the disease, and there are no states of remission. Death supervenes typically 12 to 15 years after the onset of the involuntary, jerky movements.[4] Huntington's disease is sufficiently common to provide two or three cases at any one time at the average large mental hospital. In its psychiatric aspects, Huntington's disease compares with other neurological disorders, most commonly schizophrenia. In fact, patients with Huntington's disease have been often misdiagnosed as schizophrenic psychotics or as suffering from Parkinson's disease.[5]

---

[3]The probability that a person at risk is free of the disorder increases with each symptom-free year beyond the age of 45. Nevertheless, in some at-risk persons, the disorder does not express itself until the ages of 60, 70, and even 80.

[4]There is a relatively rare juvenile form of the disorder in which definite symptoms appear before the age of 20. The downhill course in the childhood variant is rapid, characterized by severe dementia and mental depression with a suicidal tinge. The mean duration of the illness is eight years. One inexplicable aspect of the juvenile variant is that affected children, irrespective of sex, are four times more likely to have an affected father than an affected mother. See A. D. Merritt, P. M. Conneally, N. F. Rahman, and A. L. Drew, "Juvenile Huntington's chorea," *Progress in Neuro-genetics*, ed. A. Barbeau and J. R. Brunette (Amsterdam: Excerpta Medica Foundation, 1969) 645-50.

[5]Woody Guthrie, folk singer and composer, succumbed to Huntington's disease after suffering for 15 years with the disorder. His condition was initially misdiagnosed as alcoholism, for which he received little sympathy or treatment. During the last four years of his illness, he was unable to walk or talk. The persistent efforts of his wife, Marjorie Guthrie, led to the establishment of a U.S. National Commission for the Control of Huntington's Disease and Its Consequences. By focusing the spotlight on her own family, she helped to overcome the fear and intolerance of the general public to this baffling disease. See Joe Klein, *Woody Guthrie: A Life* (New York: Alfred A. Knopf, 1980).

Huntington's disease is transmitted through a single dominant gene with virtually complete penetrance. The dominant transmission means that a child need inherit only one harmful (dominant) gene, from either parent, for the disorder to appear (Plate X). A child of an affected parent has a 50-50 chance of inheriting the abnormal gene.[6] Each child has this 50 percent risk of receiving the detrimental gene irrespective of the numbers of brothers or sisters who have already shown signs of the disorder. The completeness of penetrance means that everyone who has the dominant gene ultimately will develop the disease. For the victim of Huntington's disease, the fatal determination is fixed at the moment of conception, yet the disease only becomes clinically manifest many years later. There is presently no reliable clinical or chemical test by which an affected person can be identified at an early age. If the individual knows that he or she is at risk, the years in anticipation of this dreaded disorder can be years of silent apprehension or of intense productivity.

Manifestations of the disease usually begin with personality changes, causing the patient to become irritable, moody, and irascible. The early physical signs include facial grimacing, the slurring of speech, clumsiness, and an unsteady, waddling gait. The patient experiences diminished memory and poor judgment. Both mental and physical disabilities intensify as the disorder progresses. The affected person is often plagued with fits of temper and bouts of deep depression. In the extreme condition, all parts of the body are in constant, uncontrollable motion.[7] Almost all affected persons become prematurely gray and look older

---

[6]A person affected with Huntington's disease has one mutant (dominant) gene and one normal gene (in this case, recessive). If a child of an affected parent inherits the normal (recessive) gene from both the normal parent and the affected parent, the child has not only escaped the disorder, but cannot pass it on to his or her progeny (Plate X). Huntington's disease represents but one of approximately 1,000 dominant disorders in humans in which only one abnormal (dominant) gene is necessary for the expression of the disorder. Examples of other dominant disorders are achondroplasia (disproportionate dwarfism), polydactyly (extra fingers or toes), brachydactyly (short, thick digits), and Marfan's syndrome (poor musculature and long, thin extremities). Some medical authorities believe that Abraham Lincoln, who was exceptionally long-limbed, suffered from Marfan's syndrome.

[7]There is appreciable variation in the clinical picture of Huntington's disease. In place of the characteristic choreiform movements, some patients become rigid and akinetic, and have a mask-like appearance. See D. L. Stevens, "The classification of variants of Huntington's chorea," *Advances in Neurology*, ed. A. Barbeau, J. N. Chase, and G. W. Paulson (New York: Raven Press, 1973) 1:57-64.

than their chronological age. In the final stages, there is rapid decline of intellect, a disturbance of memory, and a reduced capacity for conceptual thought. The distraught patient loses articulate speech, becomes severely emaciated (in spite of an excellent appetite), and completely loses bladder and bowel control. Death is brought on by an infection (usually pneumonia) accompanied by heart failure and muscle exhaustion. With all the devastating manifestations and the protracted downhill course to death over some 15 years, Huntington's disease is a frightful disorder for both patient and families.[8]

Attempts at treatment have been largely unsuccessful. Occupational and physical therapies remain the best means of partial relief. Drugs provide some relief for the abnormal movements and mood disturbances. Paradoxically, the disorder can virtually be eliminated in one generation if all those who now carry the gene would refrain from bearing children. However, at present, the at-risk person cannot determine his or her status until the disorder manifests itself. Because this disease most often commences in middle age, the at-risk person will usually have produced several children before knowing for certain his or her status.

The fertility of choreic persons is not at all diminished. In fact, choreics produce more children than their normal brothers and sisters. An interesting feature of this particular mutant gene is that it does not impair the reproductive fitness of the at-risk choreic while young, but such reproductive success is at the expense of bodily deterioration at a later age. A similar mutational change has been postulated as one of the primary causes of the aging process in normal individuals.[9] The mutant gene for Huntington's disease may be taken as an example of an obviously deleterious gene that could disrupt the harmony of the body at a later age, while promoting biological fitness at an earlier age.

---

[8]Given the massive long-term expenses in caring for a choreic patient, it is not unknown that the healthy spouse obtains a divorce so that the patient may qualify for medical benefits as a ward of the state.

[9]At present, there is a great deal of interest in the possibility that changes in the genetic apparatus are a strong contributing factor to aging. Aging may be due primarily to the deterioration of the genetic program that orchestrates the maintenance of cells. As time goes on, the performance of cells becomes disharmonious with the accumulation of copying errors, or mutations.

All members of the family, regardless of risk, are deeply affected by the knowledge that one or more of them may later fall prey to Huntington's disease. Mothers, in particular, have an acute premonition of which of their children will eventually succumb to the disorder. Their perception is often remarkably accurate, although not infallible. They are able to discern the increasing irritability and nervousness, the tendency toward selfishness, the decreasing lack of affection, and the withdrawal from family activities. The mother's assessment of personality changes, although subjective, are useful in alerting the physician to an incipient choreic in a family in which Huntington's disease has occurred. Physicians are still searching for a consistently reproducible clinical diagnosis. Electroencephalographic evaluations of patients do indicate a variety of minor abnormalities but fail to reveal any specific dysfunction.

Since abnormal movements are so flagrant in patients with Huntington's disease, it would seem prudent to use instruments of high sensitivity to measure motor coordination in asymptomatic individuals. Arthur Falek of the Georgia Mental Health Institute has pioneered the use of a sensitive electronic device (tremometer) to record graphically subtle motor movements of the hand of at-risk persons.[10] The preliminary results have been promising but not unequivocal. Since false positive results would have exceedingly grave consequences, it is imperative that any test to identify the genetic carrier be 100 percent diagnostic.

There is now evidence to support the hypothesis that Huntington's disease may be associated with the malfunctioning of nerve cells in the brain that respond to chemical substances known as neurotransmitters. The brain receives information, analyzes it, and then directs the appropriate response in accord with the analysis. Each junction between two nerve cells in the brain is a decisive point at which the flow of information can be inhibited, modified, or transmitted unchanged. The neurotransmitter is released across the junction between nerve cells and accordingly represents the "chemical messenger" of the brain. One prominent chemical messenger is *dopamine*, which predominates in the corpus striatum, the part of the brain associated with the coordination of motor activity.

---

[10]A. Falek and E. V. Glanville, "Investigation of genetic carriers," *Expanding Goals of Genetics in Psychiatry*, ed. F. J. Kallmann (New York: Grune & Stratton, 1962) 136-44.

Dopamine has been implicated in other neurological diseases, a good example of which is Parkinson's disease. This neurological disorder, like Huntington's disease, also produces a disturbance in motor activity, with patients showing rigidity and tremor. Parkinson patients were found to be seriously deficient in dopamine. Subsequently, these patients became dramatically improved when they were administered L-dopa, the precursor of dopamine.[11]

The major breakthrough with dopamine in the treatment of Parkinsonism brought about renewed interest in treating Huntington's disease. There was initial disappointment when it was found that the concentration of dopamine is normal in patients with Huntington's chorea. In other words, there is no deficiency of dopamine in the brain cells. This led to the speculation that the nerve cells might be hypersensitive to the available dopamine. Clinical studies have now substantiated that the nerve cells do generate a greater-than-normal response to dopamine.[12] First, the symptoms of Huntington's disease are alleviated by drugs that deplete dopamine from the brain cells, such as reserpine and tetrabenazine. Second, the clinical syndrome is attenuated when the receptors on the nerve cells are blocked from responding to dopamine by such potent neuroleptic drugs as the phenothiazines and butyrophenone haloperiodol. Finally, in contrast to Parkinson's disease, the choreiform movements in a Huntington's patient are exacerbated by L-dopa. Indeed, the L-dopa-treated Huntington patient shows psychiatric side effects that have been likened to the condition of schizophrenia.

From the foregoing observations, British scientist H. Klawans predicted that stimulation of the hypersensitive nerve receptors in asymptomatic young patients by means of L-dopa would bring out the previously undetected chorea.[13] When unaffected children in choreic families were given a large dose of L-dopa, some (but not all) developed

---

[11]A. Barbeau, "L-dopa therapy in Parkinson's disease: A critical review of nine years' experience," *Canadian Medical Association Journal* 101 (1969): 791-800.

[12]A. Barbeau, "L-dopa and juvenile Huntington's disease," *Lancet* 2 (1969): 1066; H. L. Klawans, "A pharmacologic analysis of Huntington's chorea," *European Neurology* 4 (1970): 148-63; and C. A. Soutar, "Tetrabenazine for Huntington's chorea," *British Medical Journal* 4 (1970): 55.

[13]H. C. Klawans, G. W. Paulson, and A. Barbeau, "Predictive test for Huntington's chorea," *Lancet* 2 (1970): 1185-86.

obvious facial chorea and occasional involuntary limb movements. Such abnormal signs were not witnessed in controls (normal individuals) administered L-dopa. The results only mildly suggest that the use of L-dopa might be efficacious in the recognition of the genetic carrier. The information must be viewed in a cautious vein. A positive test does not prove that the patient has Huntington's chorea. It simply indicates that the nervous system of these patients differs from the nervous system of normal persons in response to a given dose of L-dopa. A negative test is less meaningful since it is quite possible that at the time of the test the receptor sites of the nerve cells were not sufficiently altered to produce chorea. The patient may well have a negative test at one point in time and a positive test at a second trial later.

The possibility of an accurate test for the presymptomatic detection of Huntington's disease has sparked debate over the ethics of using screening techniques to detect an incurable disease.[14] The L-dopa test, if proved reliable, is not the customary type of biochemical assay in which the presence or absence of an enzyme is ascertained. It induces the actual dreaded clinical picture in the potential choreic, and as such is likely to inflict serious trauma on the individual. Some investigators firmly maintain that such a test should be withheld until something tangible, notably a cure, can be offered to those who show a positive response. The practical usefulness of the test cannot possibly compare with the psychological impact that the results would likely have on the asymptomatic person at a young age. If the test is negative, that person can have children and feel secure in the knowledge that the offspring also will be unaffected. If the test is positive, the person will doubtlessly be plunged into despondency upon learning that the only path that lies

---

[14]A discovery reported in 1983 in *Nature* represents one of the most exciting single events in current research on Huntington's disease. James Gusella and his colleagues at Massachusetts General Hospital studied two large families—one in the United States and the other in Venezuela—with extended histories of Huntington's disease. Using modern tools of DNA technology, a genetic probe (a radioactively labeled strand of DNA) has been identified that is capable of recognizing a segment of DNA closely associated with the abnormal gene for the disease. The genetic marker, or indicator, of Huntington's disease is apparently located on chromosome 4. Several questions remain to be answered before these findings can be used for predictive testing. See J. F. Gusella, N. S. Wexler, P. M. Conneally, et al., "A polymorphic DNA marker genetically linked to Huntington's disease," *Nature* 306 (1983): 234-38.

ahead in life is insidious physical and intellectual decline. The positive aspect of the test, therefore, can be worse than the current situation, which is distressful enough. At present, all offspring of parents with Huntington's disease wait anxiously throughout their lives to learn if they have been spared. All of them, however, can have some degree of optimism that they might escape, knowing the statistics give them a 50-50 chance. The test will clearly establish the ones who can *not* be optimistic about the future. Is this knowledge worse than not knowing? The critical question then is: Can an asymptomatic young person tolerate a positive response that would be provided by a reliable diagnostic test?

CHAPTER IX

SEX CHROMOSOMES, CRIMINALITY, AND MENTAL RETARDATION

Ordinarily, each person is born with two sex chromosomes: in the case of females, two X chromosomes; and in the case of males, one X and one Y. There are striking exceptions to this rule; notable among them are the few males who are born with an extra Y chromosome. These XYY males have unusually high levels of testosterone that presumably inspire overaggressiveness and antisocial behavior. This view might not have been particularly newsworthy if it had not been associated with another notion: males of XYY constitutions are prone to violence and criminality. Attributing criminal behavior to an extra Y chromosome that one inherits has resurrected the popular concept of "bad seed."[1]

---

[1] The notion that criminal behavior has an inheritable basis stems from analyses in the early 1900s of certain family histories. One prominent human "degenerate strain" was Max Jukes and his descendants. The Jukes's pedigree included over 1,000 individuals, nearly all of whom were said to be shiftless, illiterate, and intemperate. Allegedly, 130 individuals were convicted criminals, including seven murderers. Such early studies of familial predisposition to criminality are of questionable scientific validity. See R. L. Dugdale, *The Jukes: A Study in Crime, Pauperism, Disease and Heredity* (New York: Putnam's, 1910).

The effects of an extra Y chromosome on the male's behavior have touched off storms of debate that have yet to subside. The issue surfaced in 1965 when British geneticist Patricia A. Jacobs and her colleagues published their dramatic findings on the chromosomal patterns of mentally unstable inmates in a maximum security state hospital at Carstairs near Edinburgh in Scotland.[2] There was no personal contact between the patients and the investigating team so as to protect the patients' anonymity. The investigators received a coded blood sample together with a small piece of paper on which was typed the patient's date of birth, height, and psychiatric diagnosis. Jacobs was surprised to find an unusually high frequency of XYY individuals—three out of every 100 patients. Additionally, the males with two Y chromosomes were several inches taller than their XY counterparts. The suggestion was made by Jacobs that the additional sex chromosome might predispose the male to deviant behavior.

In the relatively few years since the original report, several studies have confirmed that there is a significant excess of tall XYY males in security settings.[3] Despite frequent admonitions against reaching premature conclusions, there has been a growing tendency to characterize XYY individuals as a unique group of uncontrollably aggressive psychopaths. A stereotype of the XYY male abruptly emerged: invariably tall, long limbed, having facial acne, likely to have begun criminal activity at an early age, usually with no significant family history of crime or of mental illness, and likely to resist conventional rehabilitative efforts.[4]

Several crimes of violence committed by individuals who subsequently were shown to have the XYY chromosomal constitution have received notoriety. Two widely publicized murder trials, one in France and

---

[2]P. A. Jacobs, M. Brunton, M. M. Melville, R. P. Brittain, and W. F. McClemont, "Aggressive behaviour, mental subnormality and the XYY male," *Nature* 208 (1965): 1351-52.

[3]W. M. Court Brown, W. H. Price, and P. Jacobs, "Further information on the identity of 47 XYY males," *British Medical Journal* 2 (1968): 325-31; and E. B. Hook, "Behavioral implications of the human XYY genotype," *Science* 179 (1973): 139-51.

[4]Results of a comprehensive investigation by a 12-member team indicate that the elevated crime rate of XYY males is not related to excessive aggressiveness. Although XYY males do have a higher rate of conviction for crimes than XY controls, the crimes committed were not generally acts of aggression. The criminal acts seem to be associated with lower intelligence and lower educational levels. See H. A. Witkin, S. A. Mednick, F. Schulsinger, et al., "Criminality in XYY and XXY men," *Science* 193 (1976): 547-55.

one in Australia, stand out. The 31-year-old French stablehand, Daniel Hugon, was accused of the 1965 slaying of a prostitute in a Paris hotel. After an unsuccessful suicide attempt, he was found to have an extra Y chromosome. Hugon was convicted of murder, but was given a lesser penalty on the plea of "diminished responsibility." In Melbourne, Australia, Lawrence Hannell, a 21-year-old laborer with an XYY constitution, was acquitted of murder on the strong testimony of a psychiatrist that "every cell in the defendant's brain is abnormal." The problem of understanding the nature of XYY was further compounded by the erroneous rumor that Richard Speck, the convicted murderer of eight Chicago nurses, was XYY. Tall, mentally dull, acned, with a record of 40 arrests, Speck presented the prototype of the XYY pattern. Yet, Speck did not have this chromosomal condition.

The XYY chromosomal aberration originates when the sex chromosomes are improperly distributed during the production of gametes. The double Y complement most often arises during formation of the sperm. A male normally produces two types of sperm cells—an X-bearing sperm cell and a Y-bearing sperm cell. But if the processes are abnormal, a sperm cell can arise with two Y chromosomes. When the YY sperm fertilizes a normal X-bearing egg, the outcome is an XYY male. It is estimated that 2,000 males are born in the United States each year with an XYY makeup.

The Y chromosome is one of the smallest chromosomes of the human complement and is overshadowed in size by the X chromosome. It is generally acknowledged that the larger X chromosome is the conservative partner, having undergone little change in genetic content in the course of evolution. The Y chromosome has become progressively smaller in size, and has apparently assumed an increasingly stronger role in sex determination. The Y chromosome in humans contains potent male-determining genes. An individual who carries a Y chromosome is a male, even if he has one, two, or even three X chromosomes associated with the Y.[5]

---

[5] An XY individual with an extra X is a male by virtue of the presence of the Y chromosome. Such an XXY constitution results in a sex anomaly known as "Klinefelter syndrome." Although individuals with this syndrome are male in general appearance, their testes are underdeveloped and their breasts are enlarged. The limbs of affected persons are longer than average and body hair is sparse. Many affected persons are mentally defective. The XXY disorder occurs once in every 800 liveborn males.

Since the Y chromosome carries relatively few genes, the physical abnormalities that may be present in an XYY individual would not be expected to be extensive. The physical and behavioral characteristics in XYY individuals range from apparently normal to serious impairments. As in most cases in which an extra sex chromosome is present, the genitalia are generally underdeveloped. Nevertheless, some XYY males display normal sexual development. Most XYY individuals are strikingly tall even in childhood, and usually exceed six feet in height as adults. But not all have increased stature. Facial acne appears to be frequent in adolescence, a persistent condition attributable to hormonal imbalance caused by the extra Y chromosome. Mentally, XYY individuals are usually on the borderline of the dull normal range, with IQs between 80 and 95. Nevertheless, there is a fair representation of persons with average intelligence. Abnormal electroencephalograms (EEG) have suggested some form of brain dysfunction. Yet, some XYY males with earlier findings of EEG abnormalities have later exhibited normal patterns, whereas patients with a normal EEG have later displayed abnormalities. Finally, there are males who, despite the presence of an extra Y chromosome, have displayed no unusual aggressive behavior.

The early studies were largely drawn from highly selected populations—mentally disturbed individuals and criminals in security settings. What was obviously needed were investigations of the characteristics of noninstitutionalized XYY persons in the general population. The data now available on this matter are unconvincing. The findings from some studies do suggest behavioral problems and learning disabilities in young noninstitutionalized males compared with XY controls. The XYY males are said to be more impulsive and immature than XY controls, and accordingly are presumed to be at a greater risk than XY controls for deviant behavior.[6] Other analyses do not provide evidence for a cause-effect relation between the extra Y chromosome and any behavioral problems, whether it be aggressiveness, impulsiveness, or antisocial behavior.[7] Some investigators have concluded that the as-

---

[6]B. Noel, J. B. Duport, D. Revil, I. Dussuyer, and B. Quack, "The XYY syndrome: Reality and myth," *Clinical Genetics* 5 (1974): 387-97.

[7]D. S. Borgaonkar and S. A. Shah, "The XYY chromosome male—or syndrome?" *Progress in Medical Genetics*, ed. A. G. Steinberg and A. G. Bearn (New York: Grune & Stratton, 1974) 10:135-222.

sociation between XYY males and uncontrollable excessive aggressiveness is nothing more than a myth promoted by the mass media.[8]

If there is even a slim possibility that the XYY complement is associated with deviant behavior, then a number of questions may be raised. The first is whether or not it would be desirable to undertake chromosomal analysis on all infants at birth or shortly thereafter. The expectation is that one in 1,000 newborns will have the XYY constitution. If the XYY condition can be detected at birth, are there ameliorative therapeutic measures that could be used to help XYY individuals follow less stormy lives than they might otherwise?

In 1968, a program of screening for chromosomal abnormalities in newborn males was initiated in the Boston Hospital for Women, a teaching hospital affiliated with Harvard University. The Boston study was directed by the psychiatrist Stanley Walzer and geneticist Park Gerald, both of the Harvard Medical School. These investigators believed that if the behavioral difficulties and learning disabilities could be identified early, the XYY child could be helped. Not everyone agrees. The most vocal of protagonists has been the Harvard microbiologist, Jonathan Beckwith.[9] He has objected to the chromosomal screening because of his conviction that no effective therapy, hormonal or otherwise, is possible. As Beckwith proclaims, the stigma of being XYY is so great that the behavioral problems that arise are a part of the self-fulfilling prophecy. In other words, children who are screened at birth for chromosomal abnormalities may be stigmatized by the XYY label, especially since the Y chromosome is popularly thought of as the "criminal chromosome." In essence, the upbringing of the XYY child might be distorted by parental knowledge of the abnormality, which might result in more serious problems than the abnormality might otherwise cause.

A Harvard standing committee on medical research came to the conclusion that the screening project by Walzer and Gerald was worthy of pursuit and endorsed its continuation. However, Walzer terminated the project, apparently succumbing to the criticism of Beckwith and others.

---

[8]S. Kessler and R. H. Moos, "XYY chromosome: Premature conclusions," *Science* 165 (1969): 442.

[9]J. Beckwith and J. King, "The XYY syndrome, a dangerous myth," *New Scientist* 64 (1974): 474-76; and R. Pyeritz, J. Beckwith, and L. Miller, "XYY disclosure condemned," *New England Journal of Medicine* 293 (1975): 508.

The pros and cons of XYY screening continue to be debated, but, as far as is known, there is not a single XYY newborn screening program in operation today in the United States.[10]

The human sex chromosomes continue to attract attention. In particular, the X chromosome has now been clearly shown to be involved in mental retardation. Psychologists and physicians have long recognized that mental retardation affects males more often than females. The greater vulnerability of the male apparently is associated with the X chromosome, which is paired with a Y chromosome that is largely inert genetically. Thus, a defect in the X chromosome of the male would be immediately, or overtly, expressed. In recent years, actual lesions in the X chromosome have been observed that affect the male.

In 1969, pediatrician Herbert Lubs, then at the University of Colorado Medical School, described a family in which four mentally retarded brothers each possessed an X chromosome in which the tip of the long arm appeared to be detached from the rest of the chromosome.[11] It was as if the constriction in the terminal region represented a region where the X chromosome is unusually weak or fragile.[12] This so-named "fragile X" chromosome is now known to be associated with a substantial proportion of cases of inherited mental retardation in the human male. Ironically, Lubs's report initially did not attract attention, even though the frailty of the X chromosome was most unusual.

Approximately 10 years later, the importance of Lubs's observations was appreciated. His findings were unconfirmed for several years principally because the cell culture media that most investigators subsequently used had been enriched by the addition of various growth supplements. Grant Sutherland, Adelaide Children's Hospital in Australia, discovered that only culture media deficient in folic acid and thy-

---

[10]The absence of a screening program would preclude any meaningful assessment of child-rearing behaviors of XYY males. Here, the risks of knowledge are to be weighed against the benefits, if any, of ignorance.

[11]H. A. Lubs, "A marker X chromosome," *American Journal of Human Genetics* 21 (1969): 231-44.

[12]Fragile sites have been identified in specific autosomes (particularly, 2, 10, 11, 16, and 20) when the lymphocytes are grown in certain chemically defined culture media. These chromosomal flaws are heritable, but only the fragile site in the X chromosome is associated with a clinically recognizable genetic disorder.

midine permit the expression of the fragile X site in the lymphocytes of blood.[13] Such media—deficient in certain nutrients—are now routinely used for diagnostic tests. It is ironic that the confirmation of fragile sites was set back by medical progress: the adoption in the 1970s of an enriched ("improved") culture media that actually inhibits the expression of the fragile site.[14]

In a manner that remains to be elucidated, the fragile site in the X chromosome is associated with impaired mental development in the male.[15] The most characteristic feature of the affected male, other than mental retardation, is the enlargement of the testes to several times the normal size.[16] The hormonal basis for the oversized testes ("macro-orchidism") is unclear; the levels of testosterone are normal. Additionally, affected males tend to have prominent jaws and protruding ears.

Females with retarded male sibs have been found to harbor the fragile X and some, but not all, of these carrier females have been discovered to be mildly retarded, although physically normal. A disconcerting aspect is that the fragile X chromosome is difficult to demonstrate in some female carriers. The fragile site on the X chromosome manifests itself inconsistently in carrier females, even in appropriate culture media. In particular, the fragile X is extremely difficult to demonstrate in older

---

[13]G. R. Sutherland, "Heritable fragile sites on human chromosomes. I. Factors affecting expression in lymphocyte culture," *American Journal of Human Genetics* 31 (1979): 125-35.

[14]The demonstration that folic acid inhibits the expression of the fragile site in the X chromosome has fueled ideas about preventative treatment. The suggestion has been made that mental retardation might be averted or ameliorated by supplementing the mother's diet with folic acid during pregnancy. It remains to be seen whether this idea has any merit.

[15]Not all X-linked retardation in the male is attributable to a fragile X. Among other ways, there is a recessive X-linked gene that condemns its bearers to mental retardation, cerebral palsy, and self-directed aggression. Children suffering from this "Lesch-Nyhan syndrome" compulsively mutilate themselves by biting their lips and fingers. The syndrome results from a gene-controlled absence of a single enzyme (hypoxanthine-guanine-phosphoribosyltranferase) required for normal purine metabolism.

[16]Testicular size is measured with an orchidometer, which is a series of egg-shaped beads ("Prader beads") of various volumes. Measurement is by simple visual comparison; however, the testicular volume is often greater than the largest-sized bead. The testicular volume has been found to range from 44 to 104 ml, which is several times greater than normal (10 to 25 ml).

women, those past 30 years of age.[17] Some investigators have offered the opinion that there are two forms of expression of the fragile X in the female. In one form, the carrier female exhibits no mental retardation and the appearance of the fragile site declines with the age of the carrier. In the second form, the carrier is affected mentally and invariably displays the fragile site, irrespective of age.[18]

The question then arises as to why some females are notably retarded and others are completely normal. In fact, in most X-linked diseases, a wide range of expression in the female is the general circumstance. The explanation for this phenomenon is to be found in the studies by British geneticist Mary F. Lyon in the early 1960s. She formulated the intriguing hypothesis that one X chromosome of the female becomes genetically inactive early in embryonic development and remains a muted, or silent, partner of the functional type X throughout life.[19] This "inactive X" hypothesis has become known as the Lyon hypothesis. The inactive X can be either the maternal X or the paternal X in different cells of the same female. Inactivation is thus random and independent in each cell. On the average, then, 50 percent of the paternal X chromosomes and 50 percent of the maternal X chromosomes become inactivated.

If one of the two X chromosomes is inactive, then a carrier female would be a mosaic of two populations of cells: one population with the fragile site and the other without the fragile site. A carrier female would

---

[17]The difficulties in detecting the fragile X may be illustrated by the diagnosis of a particular family with three mentally retarded brothers that was described in 1981 by a team of investigators at the University of Texas Medical School at Houston. The fragile X chromosome was found in all three retarded males, in 19 to 45 percent of their blood cells. The 57-year-old mother (who must be a carrier) had the fragile X in only three percent of her blood lymphocytes. The fragile X could not be found in one of the sisters, but was identified in 40 percent of the cells of another sister. The maternal grandmother, an obligated carrier by pedigree analysis, was 85 years old at the time of testing and did not exhibit the fragile X. See J. T. Hecht, C. M. Moore, and C. I. Scott, "A recognizable syndrome of sex-linked mental retardation, large testes, and marker X chromosome," *Southern Medical Journal* 74 (1981): 1493-95.

[18]P. N. Howard-Peebles and G. R. Stoddard, "Familial X-linked mental retardation with a marker-X chromosome and its relationship to macro-orchidism," *Clinical Genetics* 17 (1980): 125-28.

[19]There is a wealth of evidence in support of the Lyon hypothesis. Indeed, it is now quite evident that the inactivated X becomes condensed to form a cytologically conspicuous body that clings to the nuclear membrane, known as the *Barr body*.

not be affected if the normal X chromosome is functional in 50 percent or more of the cells, effectively counteracting or compensating for the fragile X chromosome in the remaining cells. However, by sheer chance, a female carrier may have a fragile X chromosome in 70 percent of her cells and the normal X in only 30 percent of the cells. In this fortuitous circumstance, the preponderance of fragile X chromosomes would be expected to cause impairment of mental ability, if only moderately.

There are still more questions than answers. These questions are likely to multiply and become even more vexing when the fragile X can be diagnosed prenatally with the use of fetal cells obtained by amniocentesis.[20]

---

[20]There are encouraging preliminary reports of the expression in amniotic cells of the fragile X chromosome. See P. B. Jacky and F. J. Dill, "Expression in fibroblast culture of the satellited-X-chromosome associated with familial sex-linked mental retardation," *Human Genetics* 53 (1980): 267-69.

CHAPTER X

PRENATAL EXPOSURE
TO HARMFUL SUBSTANCES

A variety of substances—sugar, oxygen, amino acids, and antibodies, among others—find their way across the placenta from the mother to the developing fetus. We once tacitly assumed that only beneficial substances entered the fetus. For many decades, the prevailing belief was that the fetus, sheltered in the interior of its mother, was well protected from harmful chemical or physical agents. Only in recent years has it become distressingly clear that the fetus can be injured by agents that are tolerated by, or even innocuous to, the mother. This was dramatically revealed in the early 1960s when medical researchers shockingly discovered that a supposedly harmless sleeping pill made of the drug thalidomide, when taken by the expectant mother, could lead to a bizarre defect in the child's limbs.

In 1957 a pharmaceutical firm in Stölberg, Germany, marketed a new sleeping pill made of thalidomide, which was guaranteed to provide a restful night's sleep without hangover. The manufacture of the mild sedative was licensed in other countries and within four years it became available in more than 40 countries. The sleep-inducing drug was advertised as absolutely harmless even for pregnant women, although no evidence of its safety in humans existed. Its toxic effects were soon to become apparent.

In 1959 there occurred sporadic, seemingly unrelated, cases of a peculiar deformity in newborns. The infants' arms were absent or reduced to tiny, flipperlike stumps. In some infants the legs were similarly affected; in most cases, the deformities of the legs were less severe. The external ear was sometimes malformed, and obstructive lesions of the heart and intestine were common. Mentality was normal in the vast majority of the afflicted infants. This rare condition is phocomelia, literally "seal limbs," from the Greek words *phokos* meaning "seal" and *melos* meaning "extremities."

By 1961 the incidence of phocomelia rose sharply in West Germany. In one Hamburg pediatric clinic alone, 154 cases were reported in a short span of months that year. Obstetricians sought frantically for a cause. By the end of 1961, Dr. Widukind Lenz, director of the University Clinic for Children in Hamburg, tracked down thalidomide as the one common factor in this catastrophic outbreak. All mothers of the deformed babies had taken thalidomide in the early stages of pregnancy, during the critical period in development when the infant's arms and legs were being formed.

At the 1961 pediatric meeting at Düsseldorf, Lenz reported his suspicion that thalidomide was the harmful agent. He did not name the drug in his speech, but it became quickly known among German physicians that thalidomide was the drug under suspicion.[1] Almost simultaneously, and independently, Australian pediatrician W. G. McBride gave the alarm of the crippling effects of thalidomide from the other side of the world.[2]

In November 1961 the sedative was withdrawn from the market in Germany. The United States was largely spared the thalidomide disaster by the astute scientific sense of Dr. Frances O. Kelsey of the U.S. Food

---

[1] Dr. Lenz was initially cautious in expressing his suspicions about the harmful effects of thalidomide. At the 1961 pediatric meeting, he said: "From a scientific point of view it seems premature to discuss it. But as a human being and as a citizen, I cannot remain silent about my observations." See W. Lenz, "Thalidomide and congenital abnormalities," *Lancet* 2 (1962): 45.

[2] W. G. McBride, "Thalidomide and congenital abnormalities," *Lancet* 2 (1961): 1358.

and Drug Administration who blocked general distribution of the drug. Despite her efforts, some American women did obtain it from European sources. Although relatively rare in the United States, more than 5,000 thalidomide babies were born in West Germany and at least 1,000 in other countries. The deformity was reported from widely different parts of the world—Australia, Scotland, England, Canada, Belgium, Switzerland, Lebanon, Israel, and Peru. The thalidomide tragedy changed the attitude of the medical profession toward drug-induced malformations. It also awakened the mass media; congenital defects rapidly became a subject of compelling interest to the general public.

There is scarcely any doubt that the tissues of the embryo at certain stages in differentiation are extremely sensitive to thalidomide.[3] Lenz made a careful study of the types of defects in relation to the time of intake of the drug. He determined that the sensitive period of the embryo to thalidomide fell between the 34th and 50th days after the last menstrual period (approximately the third to fourth week of embryonic life). Relatively early intake, between the 34th and 38th days, was associated primarily with gross abnormalities of the ears. Serious damage to the arms resulted when the drug had been taken between the 39th and 44th days. In most cases of deformities of the long bones of the legs, thalidomide had been taken between the 44th and 48th days. Disturbances of the intestinal tract and heart defects were common when mothers had used the drug between the 40th and 45th days. Many of the women had taken thalidomide during the period when they were unaware that they were pregnant.[4] Only one or two tablets (a single dose of 100 milligrams!) has been shown to be sufficient to cause the limb abnormality.

---

[3]The development of an organ or part may be compared to the assemblage of a car in a factory. The assembly line must move at a definite speed, as must the developmental process. At precise intervals a particular part must be attached at the proper site. If one piece is left out at a given time, all subsequent operations are hindered and the final outcome is a faulty vehicle or no car at all. Similarly, a defective gene or a noxious environmental agent may either utterly destroy the whole fabric of development or alter the synchronized processes to the extent of producing a malformed body part.

[4]A genetically determined malformation is foreordained at the time of fertilization. An environmentally determined anomaly originates from injury to the embryo at a vulnerable stage in its development. It is often quite difficult to ascertain which of the two factors—inheritance of defective genes or adverse effects of external influences—has played the major role in the appearance of the deformity. Unfavorable environmental factors may produce malformations that are similar to those resulting from a defective gene.

Expectant mothers, despite the thalidomide scare, are still consuming large quantities of drugs in the early stage of their pregnancy. The pregnant woman today in the United States consumes an average of four drugs. It should be emphasized that the unborn child has little control over the chemical environment furnished it by the mother.[5] Restraint in using drugs on the part of the pregnant woman would appear to be an exemplary virtue.

Maternal diseases such as diabetes, syphilis, tuberculosis, and German measles also represent potential danger to the developing fetus. German measles—rubella—is a relatively mild disease caused by a virus. The lymph glands behind the ears swell, rose-pink rashes develop, and a slight fever occurs. Although German measles is a disease of children, it can be contracted by adults. One out of every five persons reaches reproductive age having escaped rubella in childhood. When infection occurs in adult life, it may go undiagnosed without special laboratory tests. In other words, some adults become infected without displaying any symptoms of the disease. This is particularly unfortunate for women during their pregnancy, since the evidence is overwhelming that the rubella virus can be transmitted from the mother to the fetus. Moreover, the tissues of the fetus are more vulnerable to the viral infection than the mother's.

Moreover, an abnormal gene does not invariably produce the detrimental effect that might have been expected. Under certain environmental conditions, the defective gene may not express itself, or cause only a minor, scarcely noticeable, abnormality. One aspect is certain: the vast majority of deformities originate at an early stage of embryonic development, even before the mother may suspect that she is pregnant. The crucial period of development precedes the eighth week of pregnancy, before any visible sign is detected.

[5] Human geneticist James V. Neel estimates that approximately 20 percent of all congenital anomalies result from major defective genes with relatively simple inheritance patterns. In these cases, the genetic effects are scarcely tempered by environmental influences. Not more than 10 percent of the total can be accountable by mishaps in chromosome numbers, an intriguing phenomenon that was discussed in chapter 1. An additional 10 percent result from the action of very specific agents, such as thalidomide, in which the genetic constitution of the mother or the fetus does not appear to play a modulating role. The remaining 60 percent represents the disruption of developmental pathways occasioned by the interaction of complex genetic systems and relatively minor environmental fluctuations. Stated another way, an hereditary predisposition that might otherwise not reveal itself may be triggered to produce a malformation by subtle adverse factors in the maternal environment.

In 1940 Australia was hit by a widespread epidemic of rubella. A year after the outbreak, Australian ophthalmologist Norman McAlister Gregg drew attention to an alarming number of cases of congenital cataracts in newborn infants.[6] The lenses of the infants' eyes were opaque, obstructing the passage of light. Of 78 blinded infants, all but 10 of their mothers recalled having had German measles during the first three months of pregnancy. Gregg incriminated the rubella virus as the causative agent of the eye deformities.

History repeated itself when a severe epidemic of rubella swept across Sweden in the spring of 1951 and across the United States in the early spring of 1964. The danger to the unborn child following rubella infection became manifestly evident. The birth of defective infants was correlated with a positive history of rubella in nearly all their mothers. In the 1964 outbreak in the United States, 10,000 newborns were afflicted with cataracts. In addition, 15 percent of the pregnancies complicated by rubella terminated in spontaneous abortions or stillbirths.

The rubella virus has more than one effect on the infant. As well as being affected with cataracts, many infants are born with malformed hearts, for the most part uncorrectable. Some suffer deafness, others are mentally retarded, and still others are microcephalic (head size considerably below normal). The newborn infants are generally stunted in growth, most weighing less than 5.5 pounds and many less than 4.5 pounds at birth.

The risk of deformities in the fetus from maternal rubella is almost wholly during the first three months of pregnancy. The earlier in pregnancy that the infection occurs, the greater the chances of injury to the infant. Several studies have confirmed that about 47 percent of the newborn babies are abnormal if their mothers acquired the disease during the first month of pregnancy. The incidence of fetal defects decreases to 22 percent when maternal rubella occurs in the second month, and to seven percent in the third month. After the third month of pregnancy, the risk of fetal malformations from maternal rubella is negligible.[7]

---

[6]N. M. Gregg, "Congenital cataract following German measles in mother," *Transactions Ophthalmologist Society Australia* 3 (1941): 35-46.

[7]R. H. Michaels and G. W. Mellin, "Prospective experience with maternal rubella and associated congenital malformations," *Pediatrics* 26 (1960): 200-209.

In recent years, rubella-affected infants have become rarer. In 1969, a vaccine, made from a weakened form of the live rubella virus, was successfully developed and marketed. Its development began in 1961 when several investigators isolated the virus and devised the means of growing it in laboratory cultures. In the form of a vaccine, the weakened virus does not cause the disease, but triggers the production of protective substances, or antibodies. Antibodies, building an immunity that lasts for years, combat the virus if the person is exposed to rubella infection in later life.

With the hope of conferring immunity particularly to young women before they reach the childbearing age, a campaign was launched in 1969 to vaccinate all children between the ages of one and seven. The mass inoculations of children were also intended to prevent widespread outbreaks of the disease, or at least reduce the spread of the disease, thus minimizing the risk of exposure of pregnant women. Pregnant women themselves were not inoculated for fear that the virus, although weakened, might produce an infection of the placenta and fetal tissues.

Improper diet, obesity, excessive smoking, and alcohol may also interfere with proper development or delivery of the fetus. The deleterious effects of alcohol on the intrauterine development of the fetus are no longer debated, even though the mechanism by which alcohol produces its disturbing effects still remain unknown.[8] There is a distinctive cluster of anomalies in the offspring of mothers who consume alcohol, a pattern of defects that has been termed the "fetal alcohol syndrome." The pronounced flattened facial appearance of the affected child is as readily identifiable at birth as the characteristic face of a child with Down syndrome. The eyes are small, the nose is short and upturned, and the upper lip is underdeveloped (hypoplastic). In particular, the border of the upper lip is unusually thin, and the characteristic vertical groove in the midline is diminished or absent. Children born of chronically alcoholic women are smaller than normal, are irritable as infants, and are hyperactive as older children. On various standard performance tests (Stan-

---

[8]D. W. Smith, "The fetal alcohol syndrome," *Hospital Practice* 14 (1979): 121-28; A. P. Streissguth, S. Landesman-Dwyer, J. C. Martin, and D. W. Smith, "Teratogenic effects of alcohol in humans and laboratory animals," *Science* 209 (1970): 353-61; and C. J. Stephens, "The fetal alcohol syndrome: Cause for concern," *American Journal of Maternal Child Nursing* 6 (1981): 69-78.

ford-Binet, Bayley, or Denver scales), the affected child scores well below the normal range. Intrauterine alcohol damage may represent one of the most common causes of mental retardation in the United States today. There appears to be no minimum safe level of maternal alcohol consumption. Even moderate amounts of alcohol can have adverse effects on the developing fetus. The most prudent action would be abstinence from drinking from conception throughout the pregnancy.

Cigarette smoking during pregnancy has also been shown to affect the well-being of the fetus.[9] The concentration of carbon monoxide is abnormally high in these fetuses, which may lead to a rapid and irregular fetal heartbeat. The incidence of premature births is approximately twice as high among mothers who smoked during pregnancy as among nonsmokers. Some 4,500 stillbirths each year in the United States have been attributed to the smoking habits of pregnant women. Additionally, hospital records reveal that smokers tend to have smaller babies; the babies weigh five to eight ounces less than babies born to women who abstain from smoking during pregnancy.

Drugs may have little or no detrimental effect on the mother and yet may prove harmful to the fetus. Numerous drugs have been suspected of acting as potent *teratogens*—substances capable of causing marked developmental deviations. Current knowledge of the potential teratogenic hazards of many drugs is limited. Nevertheless, fetal malformations have been associated with tranquilizing drugs taken by the pregnant mother, such as chlorpromazine, meprobamate, and reserpine. All commonly used sulfonamides (sulfanilamide and sulfathiazole) readily cross the placenta into the fetal circulation and may have toxic effects. Barbiturates (such as sodium barbital and pentobarbital) and certain antibiotics (streptomycin, terramycin, and chloromycetin) are also possible hazards to the fetus. Behavioral traits of the offspring may be affected by the intake of certain drugs during pregnancy. Laboratory experiments have shown that the administration of the tranquilizer, meprobamate, to pregnant rats seriously interferes with the learning capacity of the offspring. In the human, adverse behavioral effects, such as speech disorders and reading difficulties in children, have been associated with

---

[9]D. S. Holsclaw, Jr., and A. L. Topham, "The effects of smoking on fetal, neonatal, and childhood development," *Pediatric Annals* 7 (1978): 201-21.

maternal complications such as eclampsia (convulsions), vaginal bleed-
ing, and premature delivery.

The controversy over the teratogenic potential of the influenza virus
may be taken as a striking demonstration of the uncertainties that exist.[10]
In the laboratory, it has been shown that chicken embryos, infected with
influenza virus, develop severe malformations such as anencephaly and
microcephaly. A high abortion rate has been witnessed in pregnant mice
infected with a human strain of influenza virus. In humans, the relation
of maternal influenza to fetal anomalies is far from clear. The pandemic
of Asian influenzia in 1957 provided an unusual opportunity for investigation. Most medical observers in the United States have argued that
there has been no significant increase in anomalies in infants born to
women who had had Asian influenza during their pregnancy. On the
other hand, investigators in Ireland have claimed a substantial increase
in fetal deformities attributable to Asian influenza. Still other investigators have asserted that the influenza virus leads to early widespread
damage of the embryo, resulting in a high incidence of abortions and
stillbirths. One cannot draw any valid conclusions, although it would be
unwarranted to conclude at this time that the influenza virus is not teratogenic in humans.

Not all cases of suspected teratogenesis can be dismissed as incon-
clusive. A synthetic hormone, diethylstilbestrol (DES), widely used to
control estrogen-deficiency disorders in women, has been recently incriminated as a cancer-inducing agent. Specifically, DES has been
strongly implicated in the occurrence of a rare form of vaginal cancer in
the daughters of women who took DES during pregnancy to prevent
miscarriages. The rare type of cancer of the genital tract appears in the
affected daughters some 15 to 22 years after exposure of the mother.
Pregnant women have been advised to avoid the use of this synthetic es-
trogen, lest their infant daughters later develop vaginal cancer.[11]

---

[10]V. P. Coffey and W. J. E. Jessop, "Maternal influenza and congenital deformities,"
Lancet 2 (1959): 935-38; M. G. Wilson, H. L. Heins, D. T. Imagawa, and J. M. Adams,
"Teratogenic effects of Asian influenza," *Journal of the American Medical Association* 171
(1959): 638-41.

[11]Recent studies have revealed structural defects in the genital tracts of males who
were prenatally exposed to diethylstilbestrol. See A. L. Herbst, H. Ulfelder, and D. C.
Poskanzer, "Adenocarcinoma of the vagina: association of maternal stilbestrol therapy
with tumor appearance in young women," *New England Journal of Medicine* 284 (1971):

Another widely publicized chemical teratogen in humans is organic mercury, a contaminant of coastal waters. Symptoms of mercury poisoning in adults, which do not appear until weeks after the ingestion of mercury-contaminated fish and shellfish, include inharmonious muscular movement, mental relapses, and loss of vision and hearing.[12] In one severe outbreak of mercury poisoning in Japan, there were 23 affected babies born to mothers who consumed large amounts of contaminated fish while pregnant. Many of the mothers were not themselves affected, but at birth, or shortly thereafter, their infants developed palsy-like symptoms (irregular movements, seizures, and marked mental retardation). Clearly, organic mercury crosses the so-called placental barrier. There is also substantial evidence that heroin and related opiates find their way across the placenta. Among infants born to heroin-dependent mothers, two out of every three manifest signs of narcotic withdrawal the first four days of life. Most of these newborn infants require drug treatment to suppress the abstinence syndrome. Behavior problems and learning difficulties have been observed in preschool children born to heroin-addicted mothers.[13]

The advent of the atomic age has focused attention on the hazards to the fetus of high energy, or ionizing, radiation. In discussing the hazards of X rays and other ionizing radiation, we must be careful to distinguish between somatic (body) damage and genetic damage. Injury to the body cells of the exposed individual constitutes somatic damage. Impairment of the genetic apparatus of the sex cells represents genetic damage. Typically the genetic alterations do not manifest themselves in the immediate individual but present a risk for his or her descendants in succeeding generations.[14]

878-81; W. B. Gill, G. F. B. Schumacher and M. Bibbo, "Structural and functional abnormalities in the sex organs of male offspring of mothers treated with DES," *Journal of Reproductive Medicine* 16 (1976): 147-53.

[12]F. Bakir, S. F. Damluji, L. Amin-Zaki, et al., "Methylmercury poisoning in Iraq: An interuniversity report," *Science* 181 (1973): 230-41; and M. Harada, "Congenital Minamata disease: intrauterine methylmercury poisoning," *Teratology* 18 (1978): 285-88.

[13]M. L. Stone, L. J. Salerno, M. Green, and C. Zelson, "Narcotic addiction in pregnancy," *American Journal of Obstetrics and Gynecology* 109 (1971): 716-23; G. S. Wilson, R. McCreary, J. Kean, and J. C. Baxter, "The development of preschool children of heroin-addicted mothers: a controlled study," *Pediatrics* 63 (1979): 135-41.

[14]The danger of irradiation is not only impairment of the body structures of the fetus, but also damage to the hereditary units (the genes) in the germinal tissues of the gonads

There are documented records of the somatic consequences of exposure to the 1945 atomic blasts in Hiroshima and Nagasaki.[15] Among 161 children born to women who were exposed to the atomic bomb while pregnant, 29 were microcephalic and 11 of these 29 were mentally retarded. As might have been expected, the detrimental effects were most pronounced among the infants of women who were in an early stage of pregnancy (less than 15 weeks' gestation) at the time of exposure. Moreover, most of the women who gave birth to deformed infants were less than 1.3 miles from the center (hypocenter) of the explosion. The adverse effects on the fetus diminished in frequency and severity as the distance from the hypocenter increased.

The findings pertaining to the atomic blasts substantiate the association found in a much earlier study between exposure to radiation and the incidence of microcephaly. The early illuminating study was carried out in 1929 by Dr. Douglas P. Murphy and his co-workers at the Department of Obstetrics of the University of Pennsylvania.[16] Among 74 newborn infants whose mothers had been administered therapeutic amounts of pelvic radium or X rays during pregnancy, 38 (50 percent) had serious defects. In 10 of these malformed infants, factors other than irradiation were implicated. In the remaining 28, the pelvic irradiation was judged to be the sole causative agent. Sixteen of the 28 infants were microcephalic and mentally retarded. This unusually high incidence of microcephaly constituted strong presumptive evidence that the anomalies were radiation-induced. Other abnormalities observed included hydrocephaly, spina bifida, and clubfoot. It is apparent that pelvic irradiation should be avoided when at all possible during pregnancy.

---

of the mother and child. Whereas radiation-induced body anomalies are not passed on to the next generation, radiation-induced defective genes can be transmitted to subsequent generations. Indeed, the concealed genetic damage can be considerable.

[15]R. W. Miller, "Delayed radiation effects in atomic-bomb survivors," *Science* 166 (1969): 569-74.

[16]D. P. Murphy, "Outcome of 625 pregnancies in women subjected to pelvic radium or roentgen irradiation," *American Journal of Obstetrics and Gynecology* 18 (1929): 179-87; and L. Goldstein and D. P. Murphy, "Microcephalic idiocy following radium therapy for uterine cancer during pregnancy," ibid., 189-95.

Studies of teratogenic agents in experimental animals in the laboratory have aided our understanding of fetal anomalies in humans. However, investigators have been quick to notice that the patterns of abnormalities may be quite different in the various species. Thus, when pregnant rats are fed a diet deficient in vitamin A, the offspring are typically hydrocephalic (enlarged head). Mice maintained on diets deficient in vitamin A during pregnancy produced offspring with ocular and kidney defects. Thalidomide in humans is a violent teratogen; yet, in testing with a wide variety of laboratory animals, thalidomide has proved to be relatively innocuous. The wide variability of response by different species reinforces the notion that the final proof of whether or not a drug is likely to be harmful to human beings must be sought in the human species itself.[17]

While indispensable information can and should be obtained from research on other animals, the effects of drugs, viruses, and other agents on embryonic tissues are often specific to human beings. This consideration would seem to mandate the use of human abortuses for experimentation. Yet, strong voices have been raised against the use in research of human embryonic and fetal tissues. In the absence of direct experimentation on aborted fetuses, is there any other way of obtaining meaningful information on human developmental abnormalities?

---

[17]The U.S. Food and Drug Administration in 1982 approved the use of the drug Accutane for the treatment of severe cases of cystic acne—a chronic disease that affects the facial oil (sebaceous) glands and can cause deep scars, physically as well as psychologically. Within the short span of a few months, numerous reports appeared of adverse effects of the drug in pregnant women. In early April 1984, the Center for Disease Control in Atlanta, Georgia, strongly advised expectant mothers to avoid the use of Accutane, as evidence continued to accumulate that this drug can induce spontaneous abortions and birth abnormalities.

CHAPTER XI

THE FETUS AS PATIENT

U ntil a few years ago, surgical intrusion into the sanctity of the womb was almost unthinkable. Physicians had accepted the futility of any effort aimed at correcting a fetal defect *in utero*. Today, dramatic progress has been made in extending medical procedures to the previously inaccessible developing fetus. The fetus is no longer a sheltered recluse, protected from outside intervention. The fetus has attained the status of a patient.

Treatment of a fetal defect *in utero* provides another option to the mother. Previously, when a disorder was diagnosed prenatally, the mother had essentially only two choices: to prepare herself for the special concerns associated with caring for a child with a birth defect, or to have an abortion. When the prenatal diagnosis forewarned of a severe handicap, the option was usually for an abortion. Now, in certain disorders, the specific malformation in the fetus not only can be recognized *in utero*, but can be managed *in utero* (Plate XI).

In 1981, a team of physicians in San Francisco, led by Dr. Michael R. Harrison, successfully operated on a congenitally obstructed urinary tract in one of a pair of unborn twins.[1] The expectant mother, Rosa Skinner, was past 40 and had elected to undergo several prenatal diagnostic tests. She learned that she was carrying twins, a girl and a boy, and that the boy had a urinary blockage. A malformation in the fetal urinary tract was readily recognizable by ultrasonography because the fluid-filled masses are conspicuous in the sonogram.[2] Had the urine continued to accumulate in the fetus, irreversible renal and pulmonary damage could have resulted. The urinary blockage almost certainly would have doomed the boy to an early death, or to a shortened life span with impaired kidneys and lungs. The obstruction of the bladder was detected about the 16th week of gestation, but surgery was not performed until the 30th week. The delay was to ensure that the normal female sibling fetus would have a chance of surviving if the surgery triggered premature delivery. A newly designed catheter was skillfully guided through the wall of Mrs. Skinner's abdomen, through the uterus, and into the distended bladder of the affected fetus. Urine was drained from the fetal abdomen into the amniotic sac. The birth of the twins took place a month early, which is not an unusual occurrence for twin deliveries. The catheter was removed, and the male twin, while requiring further corrective surgery, is expected to be as normal as his sister.

In 1983, this same team of surgeons reported the first treatment of the human fetus outside the womb. In this case, ultrasound revealed that the 21-week-old fetus had a blocked urinary tract, but the condition was too advanced to be corrected by simply inserting a catheter. The physicians made an incision into the womb, withdrew the lower half of the fetus and surgically bypassed the obstruction. The fetus was returned to the womb and carried to term. Unfortunately, the blocked uri-

---

[1]M. R. Harrison, R. A. Filly, J. T. Parer, et al., "Management of the fetus with a urinary tract malfunction," *Journal of the American Medical Association* 246 (1981): 635-39; and M. R. Harrison, M. S. Golbus, R. A. Filly, et al., "Fetal surgery for congenital hydronephrosis," *New England Journal of Medicine* 306 (1982): 591-93.

[2]The ultrasonic camera works in a manner similar to a television camera, imaging the fetus with sound waves instead of light. A urethral obstruction in the fetus is not only recognizable by ultrasonography but is commonly associated with oligohydramnios, the occurrence of less than the normal amount of amniotic fluid. The latter condition is an important indicator of functional impairment of the urinary system. See J. C. Hobbins, P. A. T. Grannum, R. L. Berkowitz, R. Silverman, M. J. Mahoney, "Ultrasound in the diagnosis of congenital anomalies," *American Journal of Obstetrics and Gynecology* 134 (1979): 331-45.

nary tract had irreversibly damaged the kidneys of the fetus and the infant died soon after birth. Nevertheless, medical surgeons remain optimistic that they can perform the same operation on other cases in time to save lives.

In a Denver hospital, another type of fetal surgery was performed in 1981. A small valve was implanted into the skull of a fetus to drain the fluid that had accumulated as a result of hydrocephalus. An accumulation of cerebrospinal fluid in the brain is a life-threatening disorder. In the absence of treatment, significant brain damage before birth can occur. Dr. William Clewell of the University of Colorado Health Sciences Center led the team that installed the valve in the 24-week-old hydrocephalic fetus.[3] The infant was delivered by caesarean section several weeks prematurely when the shunt clogged and pressure in the brain started to build again. A different type of shunt was inserted after birth.

Surgery, of course, is not always required in the prenatal treatment of the fetus. Certain inherited diseases can be treated with a large dose of vitamins or other metabolic chemicals. In 1965, physicians in Boston announced that they had successfully managed a fetus who had an inherited defect in vitamin B_{12} metabolism.[4] When the deficiency, methylmalonic acidemia, was discovered in an examination of amniotic fluid cells, large amounts of vitamin B_{12} were administered to the expectant mother. The child was born largely free of the symptoms of this rare genetic disease, and is presently developing normally on a restricted protein diet.

It would seem that prenatal therapy will take its place as an important new tool in the treatment of fetal disorders. One clearly affirmative aspect is that prenatal therapy provides an alternative to abortion. Surgical intervention is intended to improve the fetus' chances for a healthy existence. However, this hopeful prospect cannot ignore the possibility

---

[3] W. H. Clewell, M. L. Johnson, P. R. Meier, et al., "A surgical approach to the treatment of fetal hydrocephalus," *New England Journal of Medicine* 306 (1982): 1320-25.

[4] M. G. Ampola, M. J. Mahoney, E. Nakamura, and K. Tanaka, "Prenatal therapy of a patient with vitamin-B_{12}-responsive methylmalonic acidemia," *New England Journal of Medicine* 293 (1975): 313-17.

that treatment might be unsuccessful.[5] No assurance can be given to the expectant mother that the fetal ailment can be cured and that the baby will be born healthy. In the event of failure of fetal surgery, a woman who initially was prepared to abort may then have to face a baby whose life remains compromised because of unsuccessful fetal therapy.

It may be, then, that the likelihood of fetal therapy only serves to make the expectant mother's decision even more agonizing. What burden of guilt would a woman bear if she refused to allow her abnormal fetus to be treated for fear of failure of therapy? Is it morally unacceptable to allow a fetus with a treatable defect to be born without the benefit of therapy? Would it be wrong if the woman elected an abortion, even though the fetal defect could possibly be corrected? Obviously, fetal therapy has discomforting overtones. Prior to such techniques, there were only two options—abortion or the birth of a defective child. Does fetal surgery place a lid on both options? If it is morally reprehensible to allow a fetus with a treatable defect to be born without the benefit of treatment, is this tantamount to saying that only one option remains—treatment?

Are there other approaches currently available for alleviating genetic disorders? During the past several years, few scientific subjects have attracted as much widespread attention as has the masterly technology of *recombinant DNA*, or *gene-splicing*.[6] When first introduced, the novel technique evoked heated debate over its possible perils, but the controversy has largely subsided. Gene-splicing is currently acknowledged as one of our most powerful tools for revolutionizing the treatment of disease. The technique of gene-splicing involves the manipulation of the hereditary apparatus of one of nature's simplest organisms—a bacterial cell—in such a fashion that it can carry genes from very distantly related organisms, including viruses, frogs, and rabbits. The altered, or "en-

---

[5]W. R. Barclay, R. A. McCormick, J. B. Sidbury, M. Michejda, and G. D. Hodgen, "The ethics of in utero surgery," *Journal of the American Medical Association* 246 (1981): 1550-55; and W. Ruddick and W. Wilcox, "Operating on the fetus," *Hastings Center Report* 12 (1982): 10-14.

[6]J. D. Baxter, "Recombinant DNA and medical progress," *Hospital Practice* 15 (1980): 57-67; W. Gilbert and L. Villa-Komaroff, "Useful proteins for recombinant bacteria," *Scientific American* 242 (1980): 74-94; and W. L. Miller, "Recombinant DNA and the pediatrician," *Journal of Pediatrics* 99 (1981): 1-15.

gineered," bacterial cell has the capability of producing biologically important substances, such as antibodies and hormones. The microbe that has played the major role in the gene-splicing process is the rod-like bacterium known as *Escherichia coli*, a normal inhabitant of the human intestine and usually harmless.

The hereditary apparatus of the *coli* bacterium is virtually unique among organisms. The bacterial cell has a large circular strand of deoxyribonucleic acid (DNA) that contains several hundred genes.[7] In addition, there are several smaller loops of DNA called plasmids, which carry from two to 250 genes, depending on the size of the ring (Plate XII). A plasmid can be isolated in pure form from the bacterium and experimentally fragmented at specific points. The experimental cleaving of plasmids has been made possible by the discovery of a class of enzymes called *restriction endonucleases*. These enzymes act as chemical scissors; they cut the plasmid DNA at precise sites.

The DNA molecule from the cell of another organism—an insect, a frog, or a mouse, for example—can be removed and portions of this DNA molecule can be isolated by the use of restriction enzymes. This isolated strip of genetic information can then be inserted, or "spliced," into the gap of the open plasmid loop. The outcome is a new DNA circle, or a recombinant DNA molecule (Plate XII). The "snip-and-fit" procedure may be compared to the manner in which a jeweler expands a ring—a small piece of metal obtained from another ring is cemented into place in the gap of the forcibly opened ring.

The newly formed recombinant DNA molecule, when reintroduced into a bacterium, can duplicate itself precisely and be passed to daughter bacterial cells for many generations. In simple terms, the new DNA molecule can be manufactured in unlimited quantities as the bacteria repro-

---

[7]One of the finest triumphs of modern science has been the elucidation of the chemical nature of the gene. The transmission of traits from parents to offspring depends on the transfer of a specific giant molecule that carries a coded blueprint in its molecular structure. This complex molecule, the basic chemical component of the chromosome, is *deoxyribonucleic acid*, referred to in its abbreviated form, DNA. The information carried in this molecule can be divided into a number of separable units, now recognized as the genes. Stated simply, chromosomes are primarily long strands of DNA, and genes are coded sequences of the DNA molecule. The amount of DNA present in a single unfertilized human egg has been estimated to carry information corresponding to two million genes.

duce in their usual prolific manner. This ingenious technique thus permits the large-scale transmission of genes that code for indispensable proteins and hormones. As a striking example, the insertion of the insulin-producing gene of the laboratory rat into *Escherichia coli* has made possible the production of invaluable insulin in large quantities.[8] The limitless availability of biosynthetic insulin will effectively eliminate the shortages of bovine insulin and will make it possible for all children with diabetes to be treated. Tests with human volunteers in Great Britain have shown that the biosynthetic insulin is safe to use.

One of the outstanding successes of the gene-splicing approach has been the production of human growth hormone.[9] In this case, the genes coding for the proteins of the growth hormone were actually synthesized chemically in the laboratory. The synthetically created genes were incorporated into *Escherichia coli* and efficient synthesis of human growth hormone was achieved. Tests have already been initiated on children in several medical centers with the artificial growth hormone produced by recombinant bacteria. The growth hormone is used to treat pituitary dwarfs and may be valuable in treating burns and healing broken bones.

In addition to human growth hormone and insulin, other valuable proteins such as ovalbumin and interferon have been produced by recombinant DNA technology. Interferon, a chemical produced by the human body to ward off viruses, has been hailed as a wonder drug to combat cancer. Since this chemical substance is specific to humans, it is not obtainable from laboratory or domestic animals. Moreover, interferon exists only in minute amounts in the human body. The gene-splicing procedure has made large quantities of interferon available for use in experimental trials. The therapeutic value of interferon in the treatment of human cancers is still unknown, notwithstanding the heightened expectations generated by the mass media.

The recombinant DNA technology has permitted the development of a safer and more sensitive procedure for the prenatal diagnosis of sickle

---

[8]A. D. Riggs, "Bacterial production of human insulin," *Diabetes Care* 4 (1981): 64-68; and I. S. Johnson, "Human insulin from recombinant DNA technology," *Science* 219 (1983): 632-37.

[9]J. H. Martial, R. A. Hallewell, J. D. Baxter, et al., "Human growth hormone: Complementary DNA cloning and expression in bacteria," *Science* 205 (1979): 602-607.

cell anemia.[10] This disease is associated with a gene that codes for a polypeptide chain (the *beta* chain) of the hemoglobin molecule (see chapter 4). A particular restriction enzyme (designated Hpa I) recognizes the coding sequence in the DNA molecule that is responsible for the pattern of linked amino acids in the beta polypeptide chain. In a person with normal hemoglobin, the fragment of DNA associated with the normal beta gene has a characteristic length. In contrast, the strand of sickle cell DNA cleaved by the restriction enzyme is typically longer than normal.[11] Accordingly, since the defective gene in sickle cell DNA does not generate the same, normal pattern of amino acids, the DNA fragments that are cleaved by the restriction enzyme are different—in this case, longer. The technique is so sensitive that cells from just 15 ml of amniotic fluid are sufficient to make the diagnosis.

The recombinant DNA technique promises new ways of remedying human disease. Eventually it may be possible to insert a normal gene into the cells of a patient suffering from an inborn error of metabolism with the intent of overcoming the adverse effects of the mutant gene. Thus, it is likely that investigators will be able to splice into a bacterial cell a sequence of DNA bases that specifies the production of the enzyme, phenylalanine hydroxylase, which is deficient or absent in PKU patients. The carrier bacteria can then be introduced, and, it is hoped, integrated, into the cells of a newborn infant (or even fetus), with the expectation that the donor-DNA sequence will promote the production of the enzyme that is errant in the patient. Ideally, the recombinant DNA should be inserted only in liver cells, which are the only cells in the body that normally exhibit phenylalanine hydroxylase activity. In an effort to ensure that the new gene is placed in the proper target cells, the liver cells could be obtained by biopsy from patients with phenylketonuria. Then,

---

[10]Y. W. Kan and A. M. Dozy, "Antenatal diagnosis of sickle-cell anaemia by D.N.A. analysis of amniotic-fluid cells," *Lancet* 2 (1978): 910-12.

[11]Three types of fragments bearing the gene that codes for the beta chain of hemoglobin are produced by digesting human DNA with the restriction enzyme Hpa I. The lengths of the fragments are delineated in kilobases (kb). The normal beta gene is located on a DNA fragment that is either 7.0 or 7.6 kb (7,000 or 7,600 nucleotides) in length. In contrast, the aberrant beta (sickle cell) gene is located on a fragment that is 13 kb long. This gene is associated with the loss of a recognition site for the restriction enzyme with the outcome that a larger than normal fragment (13 kb rather than 7.0 or 7.6 kb) is produced when the sickle cell DNA is cleaved.

after the normal phenylalanine hydroxylase gene is inserted, the liver cells could be reimplanted.

Another approach to the alleviation of inherited disorders is the transplantation of tissues and organs from one individual to another. When bone marrow is transplanted, the transplanted blood cells colonize in the host's marrow in the long bones, multiply in these sites, and produce blood cells that are characteristic of the donor. Moderate success has been attained in injecting normal marrow cells into human patients suffering from *agammaglobulinemia*, a disorder characterized by a deficiency or lack of antibodies. Ultimately, the transplantation of healthy donor tissues may prove to be the most important way of controlling or curing many genetic diseases of blood cells such a sickle cell anemia, hemophilia, and thalassemia.[12]

It is clear that science's newly found ability to insert spliced or recombined DNA molecules into a living cell or organism provides a unique approach to a variety of important medical problems. Nevertheless, scary scenarios of the potential hazards of DNA technology continue to bubble restlessly to the surface. The main fears revolve around the real, or fancied, danger of producing a previously unknown disease-producing bacterial strain that might spread uncontrollably to produce a devastating epidemic, or a bacterial strain that might increase the susceptibility of the human host to cancer or some other dread disease.[13] Fortunately, the sporadic alarms have abated with the realization that the

---

[12]Thalassemia represents a heterogeneous group of inherited blood diseases, often fatal, in which a globin protein is missing entirely or is produced in abnormally small quantities. Although not a major public health problem in the United States, the disease is prevalent in the Mediterranean area and in the Middle and Far East. Recent technical advances have enabled researchers to describe the molecular basis of the thalassemias in incredible detail, including sophisticated methods for the prenatal detection of certain forms of thalassemia. See S. H. Orkin, B. P. Alter, C. Altay, et al., "Application of endonuclease mapping to the analysis and prenatal diagnosis of thalassemias caused by globin-gene deletion," *New England Journal of Medicine* 299 (1978): 166-72; A. M. Dozy, E. N. Forman, D. N. Abuelo, et al., "Prenatal diagnosis of homozygous α-thalassemia," *Journal of the American Medical Association* 241 (1979): 1610-12; and M. Pirastu, Y. W. Kan, A. Cao, et al., "Prenatal diagnosis of β-thalassemia," *New England Journal of Medicine* 309 (1983): 284-87.

[13]C. Grobstein, *A Double Image of the Double Helix* (San Francisco: W. H. Freeman and Company, 1979); and D. A. Jackson and S. P. Stich, eds., *The Recombinant DNA Debate* (New Jersey: Prentice Hall, 1979).

hazards have been quite exaggerated. One way of limiting possible dangers has been the establishment of very careful guidelines for research in DNA technology. The guidelines do not compromise the previous freedom of scientific inquiry, but they do provide the public with a measure of protection that goes beyond the mere promise of scientists to be watchful.[14] Although the risks are more imagined than real, careful observance of the guidelines will continue to be necessary to insure that this remarkable new technology is used for the maximum potential good.

---

[14]In 1980, hematologist Martin Cline of the University of California at Los Angeles used a modified form of gene-splicing in an endeavor to cure two women, one in Israel and one in Italy, of the fatal blood disease, *beta*-thalassemia. Cline undertook the experimental trials abroad where regulations are less restrictive. Marrow cells from each patient were removed, and DNA sequences containing the appropriate gene for normal globin synthesis were placed adjacent to the marrow cells in a test tube. Later, when some of the patient's marrow cells might have incorporated the normal globin gene, the marrow cells were re-introduced into the patient. There were no beneficial effects in either woman. Cline was severely reprimanded by the scientific community for the premature application of an experimental technique. In another decade, Cline may well be seen as a pioneer, however ill-advised his untimely action is viewed today.

CHAPTER XII

THE "TEST-TUBE" BABY

On the 25th of July 1978, banner headlines in Britain announced that a 30-year-old woman in a northern English textile town had given birth to a daughter who had begun life as a fertilized egg in a laboratory culture dish. In journalistic vernacular, the world was said to have witnessed its first "test-tube" baby. It is more accurate to say that society took notice of an extraordinary series of events: a human egg was recovered from a woman's ovary, fertilized in glassware (*in vitro*) by sperm from the husband, grown in a culture medium until an appropriate stage for implantation, when it was then transferred to the woman's uterus where it developed to term.

The 30-year-old mother was Lesley Brown, childless after nine years of marriage because of a blockage in her fallopian tubes. On that memorable day in July, Mrs. Brown gave birth during a 45-minute caesarean operation to a 5-pound, 12-ounce girl, nine days premature. The delivery of Louise Joy Brown in Oldham General Hospital was made possible by the ideal working relationship of two scientists—Patrick Steptoe, a highly respected gynecologist, and his colleague, Robert Edwards, a well-known Cambridge University physiologist. This remarkable breakthrough was first reported sketchily in the 12 August 1978 issue of the medical journal *Lancet*, and became the absorbing topic of discussion at several meetings of clinical societies in 1979.[1]

Shortly after the dramatic event, gynecologists were besieged with calls from countless numbers of infertile women demanding the technique, as if the procedures were already routine, faultless, and blameless. Newspapers throughout the world carried stories of women clamoring for the "miracle." Most people were exceptionally naive about the procedures. Incredibly, many persons conjured images of bubbling test tubes and even electric sparks molding the embryo into shape. It bears emphasizing that the "test-tube" baby is not a laboratory baby. Indeed, the baby spent only a very brief portion of its nine-months' existence outside the womb of the mother.

To bypass the defect in Lesley Brown's fallopian tubes, Steptoe and Edwards undertook an elaborate procedure that they had developed over a ten-year period (Plate XIII). Using a surgical technique called laparoscopy, they removed a mature egg (oocyte) from Mrs. Brown's ovary just before ovulation was expected. A clear view of the ovary was obtained with a slender illuminated telescope, laparoscope, that was inserted through a small incision made in the abdominal wall. A specially designed hypodermic needle was then passed through a small slit in the abdomen, and the egg of the bulging follicle was aspirated.[2] The

---

[1]The birth of Louise Joy Brown was discussed in a brief communication on 12 August 1978 by P. C. Steptoe and R. G. Edwards (*Lancet* 2 [1978]: 8080). In January 1979, the team of investigators delivered a series of instructive lectures before the Royal College of Obstetricians and Gynecologists. These lectures appeared in print in 1980. See R. G. Edwards, P. C. Steptoe, and J. M. Purdy, "Establishing full-term human pregnancies using cleaving embryos grown *in vitro*," *British Journal of Obstetrics and Gynaecology* 87 (1980): 737-56; P. C. Steptoe, R. G. Edwards, and J. M. Purdy, "Clinical aspects of pregnancies established with cleaving embryos grown *in vitro*," ibid., 757-68; and R. G. Edwards, P. C. Steptoe, R. E. Fowler, and J. Baillie, "Observations on preovulatory human ovarian follicles and their aspirates," ibid., 769-79.

[2]The maturation of a follicular egg may be stimulated artificially by the injection of pituitary hormones, technically called gonadotropins. First, a hormone known as human menopausal gonadotropin (HMG) is injected. This hormone, obtained from postmenopausal women, is rich in follicle-stimulating hormone (FSH). This initial injection is followed by human chorionic gonadotropin (HCG), which is remarkably similar to luteinizing hormone (LH). The luteinizing hormone normally triggers the release of the egg from the bulging Graafian follicle. Steptoe and Edwards recovered the egg from the protruding follicle about four hours before the expected time of ovulation. They eventually abandoned the foregoing technique of inducing ovulation and relied on the natural hormonal cycle of the woman to recover the mature egg.

rounded follicle (containing the egg) was readily detectable on the surface of the ovary as a thin-walled pink swelling.

The extracted egg was placed in an appropriate culture medium to which was added a concentrated sperm suspension from her husband, produced by masturbation just prior to laparoscopy. In addition to the customary procedure of examining the sperm microscopically to assure that they were active, the semen was analyzed for the presence of pathogenic bacteria. Appropriate antibiotic treatment was used to destroy the harmful bacteria. After the fertilized egg had developed to a certain stage, the embryo was implanted in Lesley Brown's uterus, where it grew into a normal fetus. The placement of the embryo into the uterus was accomplished without anesthesia and just a minimum of discomfort.[3]

Normally, it takes the fertilized egg nearly a week to find its way into the wall of the uterus. Four or five days are spent journeying through the fallopian tube, during which time the egg has divided several times. The successive divisions of the egg are referred to as cleavages. After several cleavages, the embryo—no longer an egg—consists of a solid ball of cells resembling a mulberry. The embryo floats free in the uterine cavity for two or three days before invading and burrowing into the uterine wall. At the time of implantation, the embryo resembles a hollow sphere and is called a *blastocyst* (Plate III).

In September 1970, Edwards and his co-workers announced in the English journal *Nature* that several *in vitro* fertilized eggs had developed normally as far as the 16-cell stage.[4] This was followed by a published report in the January 1971 issue of *Nature* that the human embryo could be cultured to the blastocyst stage, at which point it would naturally implant itself in the uterus.[5] Initially, it was anticipated that the best out-

---

[3]In the numerous cases, the embryos were implanted in the uteri of women at varying times of the 24-hour day. Ironically, all successful pregnancies ensued when the embryos were inserted during the late evening. Since this phenomenon may represent an important instance of a biological rhythm in humans, Steptoe and Edwards invariably carried out the implantation only during the evening hours, and not during morning or afternoon hours.

[4]R. G. Edwards, P. C. Steptoe, and J. M. Purdy, "Fertilization and cleavage *in vitro* of preovulator human oocytes," *Nature* (London) 227 (1970): 1307-1309.

[5]P. C. Steptoe, R. G. Edwards, and J. M. Purdy, "Human blastocysts grown in culture," *Nature* 229 (1971): 132-33.

come would be achieved if the *in vitro* embryos were transferred at the blastocyst stage. However, studies performed on the probability of pregnancy following the placement of embryos in various stages of cleavage showed that the highest frequency of pregnancies occurred when the embryos were transferred at the 16-cell stage.

When it was established that pregnancy had occurred, Mrs. Brown was sent home and encouraged to live a normal but restful life. She returned to Oldham General Hospital for a series of tests throughout the pregnancy, staying in the hospital for two or three days on each occasion. She was examined periodically by ultrasonic scan; amniocentesis under ultrasound scrutiny was performed at approximately 16 weeks of gestation. The amniotic cells were harvested for chromosomal analyses. As reported by Steptoe and Edwards, the analyses "revealed normal alpha-fetoprotein levels, with no chromosome abnormalities in a 46 XX fetus."

The birth of Louise Brown immediately brought into focus a number of ethical issues. Concern was voiced that the procedure of *in vitro* fertilization and the subsequent transfer of the blastocyst into the uterus involves too great a risk. One cannot assess or predict whether or not the resulting infant—if it should survive—would be deformed because of the experimental manipulations. Steptoe and Edwards have contended that the benefits outweigh the risks. The dual techniques of *in vitro* fertilization and embryo transfer provide a means of overcoming a form of female infertility in which the fallopian tubes are occluded or blocked.[6] Blocked or abnormal oviducts account for approximately 20 percent of the cases of infertility in women. These techniques can also be helpful to those women who fail to conceive because the chemical fluids in the cervical canal have deleterious effects on the sperm. Additionally, some men suffer from low sperm counts, and the *in vitro* fertilization proce-

---

[6]A survey of unmarried women ages 18 to 23 randomly selected from counties adjacent to Stanford University Medical Center in California showed that 90 percent of the women would condone artificial insemination of their own egg by their husband's sperm if it were the only way they could conceive once they were married. However, when they were asked to consider artificial insemination that involved another male's sperm, or *in vitro* fertilization that involved another female's egg, the percentages dropped dramatically to 14 and 11 percent, respectively. See W. B. Miller, "Reproduction, technology, and the behavioral sciences," *Science* 183 (1974): 149.

dure requires fewer sperm cells compared with the massive numbers needed naturally.[7]

In the United States, almost all research with human eggs came to an abrupt halt in 1975. Under a 1975 federal order, the Department of Health, Education, and Welfare was barred from funding any project involving *in vitro* fertilization unless it was first approved by a national ethics advisory committee appointed by the HEW secretary. No such national advisory committee was appointed until the birth of Louise Brown.

In July of 1978, spurred by the birth of Britain's "test-tube" baby, the then HEW secretary, Joseph A. Califano, called for a national debate on whether the U.S. should finance research that could lead to a similar birth in the United States. The composition of HEW's advisory board was mixed: lawyers, obstetricians, gynecologists, medical ethicists, and businessmen.[8] Califano stated that research in reproductive biology not only would enable many childless women to bear children, but might produce knowledge that could help doctors reduce genetic diseases. He hastened to add that the novel procedures raise serious moral questions. A comprehensive, 958-page report was prepared by the advisory board in 1979. However, Congress has continued to ignore the now four-year-

---

[7]An estimated 600,000 women across the United States are unable to conceive. The American Fertility Society, Birmingham, Alabama, provides the following statistics concerning fertility: (1) one in six couples of childbearing age has a fertility problem; and (2) 40 percent of the infertility is attributable to men, 40 percent to women, and 20 percent to unknown factors.

[8]The members of the Ethics Advisory Board of the Department of Health, Education, and Welfare were as follows: James C. Gaither, San Francisco lawyer, chairman; David A. Hamburg, president, Institute of Medicine of the National Academy of Sciences, vice-chairman; Sissela Bok, lecturer, Medical Ethics, Harvard University; Jack T. Conway, senior vice-president, United Way of America; Henry W. Foster, chairman, Obstetrics and Gynecology Department, Meharry Medical College; Donald A. Henderson, dean, School of Hygiene and Public Health, Johns Hopkins University; Maurice Lazarus, executive, Federated Department Stores, Inc.; Richard A. McCormick, professor, Christian Ethics, Kennedy Institute for the Study of Reproduction and Bioethics; Robert F. Murray, chief, Medical Genetics Division, Howard University College of Medicine; Mitchell W. Spellman, dean, Medical Services, Harvard University Medical School; Daniel C. Tosteson, dean, Harvard University Medical School; Agnes N. Williams, Potomac, Maryland, lawyer; and Eugene M. Zweiback, Omaha, Nebraska, surgeon.

old recommendation to provide federal funds to support clinical trials in human *in vitro* fertilization and embryo transfer.[9]

Notwithstanding the absence of federal support, the birth of America's first "test-tube" baby was reported in late 1981. On 28 December 1981, in Norfolk, Virginia, normal 5-pound, 12-ounce Elizabeth Jane Carr was delivered by caesarean section to Judith Carr, a 28-year-old Westminster, Massachusetts, schoolteacher. The conception and birth were supervised by Drs. Howard and Georgeanna Jones at the Eastern Virginia Medical School. There are now close to two dozen "test-tube" babies in the United States, and some 150 throughout the world, mainly in Australia and the United Kingdom.[10] Not all reports of children born after embryo transfer have been substantiated.[11]

---

[9]The report of the HEW Ethics Advisory Board stressed the desirability of additional research. Identification of the normality of *in vitro* fertilized human eggs was considered one of the more critical problems. Few investigators have studied the *in vitro* development of human eggs, and even fewer have compared the products cytologically with normal human morulae or blastocysts recovered from women. Additionally, little is known of the specific characteristics and behavior of spermatozoa in artificial insemination. There is no question that, *in vivo*, the female reproductive tract plays an active role in sperm selection, transport, and capacitation—all phenomena that cannot yet be duplicated *in vitro*. The report of the advisory board proposed a detailed study of the chromosomal configurations of human embryos produced in culture to determine whether or not the chromosomal complements are statistically different from those of embryos produced *in utero*.

[10]Lesley Brown also has the distinction of being the first woman to have given birth to two children conceived by the *in vitro* fertilization technique. The mother of the world's first "test-tube" baby (Louise Joy) delivered her second child, Natalie Jane, at Bristol maternity hospital on 15 June 1982.

[11]In 1974, D. C. Bevis, apparently having used the procedures described by Edwards and Steptoe, reported in the *British Medical Journal* (vol. 3, p. 238) the birth of three children who were "apparently normal, were alive in the United Kingdom and Western Europe after embryo transplantation." Most investigators have not been convinced of the validity of Bevis's claim, as scrupulous details of his work have yet to be presented to the scientific community. In a comparable situation, Mukherjee and Bhattacharya of India reported in the *Medical World News* (25 December 1978) that they had induced superovulation in an infertile woman and had recovered five eggs, which were subsequently fertilized *in vivo*. "When the fertilized eggs reached the morula stage—8 to 22 cells— they were frozen in liquid nitrogen" and maintained in this state for 53 days before they were placed at intervals in the mother's uterus. A baby girl was reported as the successful outcome of these procedures. There has been no documentation or verification of this alleged triumph.

The achievements in the United Kingdom, Australia, and the United States do not obliterate the serious ethical concerns. In rabbits and mice, the total probability of success in withdrawing an egg from an ovarian follicle, completing *in vitro* fertilization, and obtaining a live offspring after embryo transfer is only 25 percent. To enhance the probability of success in humans, several preovulatory eggs are taken from the prospective mother for *in vitro* fertilization. When only one of several artificially fertilized eggs is implanted, who decides what is to be done with the surplus embryos? Who is responsible for destruction of the surplus specimens? Is such destruction of embryos a matter of moral indifference?

The foregoing questions might become less thorny if the surplus embryos were to be routinely frozen.[12] Recently, medical scientists in Australia have used a frozen human embryo to produce what appears to be a successful pregnancy. Dr. Alan Trounson and his colleagues at Queen Victoria Medical Center in Melbourne had induced the prospective mother to release several preovulatory eggs simultaneously. Four of the eggs had been fertilized with her husband's sperm in the laboratory, and one embryo had been implanted in her uterus. The other three were frozen in liquid nitrogen for storage. The woman suffered a miscarriage after eight weeks of pregnancy with the original embryo. At that point, one of the embryos that had been frozen was thawed and implanted. The second pregnancy has proceeded normally.

For philosophers and theologians, as well as scientists, the technique sharpens long-standing religious questions. For some theologians, *in vitro* fertilization is applauded as a humanizing technique, allowing some infertile couples the profound and worthy satisfactions of procreation and parenthood. For other theologians, the technique is another dehumanizing step toward subverting our sense of mystery and reverence for life. The Vatican reiterates the Church's long-standing position that interference with nature in any form is not acceptable. The Papacy condemns artificial insemination, even with the husband as donor.

---

[12]Several kinds of animals—mice, rats, rabbits, cattle, and sheep—have been raised from embryos that were frozen and stored for extended periods of time. In some cases, as in cattle, the embryos have been frozen for at least eight years. The frozen embryos, after thawing, have been successfully implanted in foster mothers.

The ethical questions can only become more urgent as technical capabilities provide new alternatives. Prior to implantation, small cellular fragments of the blastocyst can be excised and diagnosed for the identification of sex, chromosomal abnormalities, and biochemical defects. Would the use of the technique for selecting the offspring's sex be condoned?[13] In fact, in the case of Mrs. Brown, her baby's sex was determined in advance from chromosomal tests. Mrs. Brown did not wish to be informed because, in her words, "I don't want to be cheated of the final thrill." Do the new technologies subvert our sense of mystery?[14]

A strong argument for not endorsing *in vitro* conception is the fear of birth deformities. It has been argued that it is morally impermissible because of the greater risk that the implanted embryo will abort or be born defective. This argument does not withstand scrutiny. We know that 99.4 percent of the chromosomal abnormalities in fetuses are eliminated naturally through spontaneous abortion (chapter 2). We can reasonably expect a comparable elimination of abnormal embryos in pregnant women utilizing the technique of embryo transfer. There is no reason to

---

[13]It is clear that preselection of gender can be accomplished by amniocentesis. Some social scientists have commented on the social implications of gender preselection and its acceptance by people. Surveys have indicated that one out of three couples would select the sex of their children, given the opportunity.

[14]There is also the argument that *in vitro* fertilization and embryo transfer should be stopped now for fear of what medical scientists will do next. This "fear of the future" is an argument that has been advanced against every innovation since the discovery of fire. There is no reason to anticipate the misuse of the new technologies. Yet, there remain ill-defined apprehensions that medical scientists will create in the future a so-called chimera—one person created out of two embryos. That remarkable feat has already been accomplished in the laboratory mouse.

In the 1960s, Beatrice Mintz of the Cancer Institute of Philadelphia fused the cleavage cells derived from two different mouse embryos. The resulting single embryo thus had four parents. In this operation, the tough zona pellucida membranes of two embryos in the blastula stage are disrupted, or dissolved, by the protein-splitting enzyme, pronase. The two denuded blastulae are then placed in contact in a culture medium. The cells from each blastula unite randomly to form a composite sphere that becomes a single blastocyst. This quadriparental blastocyst is then surgically implanted in the uterus of a foster mother where it develops normally. Many of these embryos have grown into healthy, fertile adults. The first viable quadriparental mouse of this kind was born in 1965. Since then, some 500 normal animals have been experimentally produced, and many have lived a full life span. They, in turn, have left more than 25,000 offspring.

believe that the technique of embryo transfer will promote or enhance the survival of embryos with chromosomal abnormalities.[15]

There has been appreciable speculation on the ways that people in our society might use the new reproductive technologies. There are women who are capable of carrying a fetus to term, but are unable or unwilling to supply an egg. This might include women who are known carriers of an X-linked genetic disorder, such as hemophilia, or women who are at risk for late-onset dominant disorders, such as Huntington's chorea. Ultimately, a small number of women may wish to mother a child who is the product of an egg donated by another woman. "Ovum donation" (O.D.) would be the counterpart to "artificial insemination by donor" (A.I.D.).

Our society may find unpalatable the notion of using an egg from a strange donor. In this respect, it is of particular interest that society today sanctions adoption of children, and the adoptive parents rarely have knowledge of the true (biological) mother and father of the adopted child. At least one ethicist has cogently commented that essentially only one new feature is introduced by the new technologies—the younger age of the child to be adopted. When the situation is viewed in this manner, a couple, rather than adopt a grown child, could choose to accept an early blastocyst that could grow in the woman's womb.

Some women may be physically incapable of carrying a fetus to term. Cardiac disorders, partial paralysis, a history of miscarriages, or a variety of other medical disorders suggest that women who wish to be genetic parents will enlist the aid of "surrogate" mothers. In other words, a woman seeks out a substitute, or surrogate, mother for implantation of her embryo. Surrogate motherhood raises many issues. Let us assume that a couple contracts a surrogate woman to carry their fetus to term. May the couple place restrictions on the habits, the medical care, or the

---

[15]Let us assume that the treatment associated with embryo transfer does enhance the survival of naturally occurring chromosomal abnormalities. A *marked* increase in the frequency of chromosomal abnormalities at implantation is expected to have only a *minor* effect on the frequency of abnormalities among live births. Since only 0.6 percent of the abnormalities at implantation occur in fetuses that survive to the point of live birth, a twofold increase in the frequency of abnormalities at implantation, from 500 to 800 per 1,000, would result in only two to three additional abnormalities per 1,000 live births.

diet of the surrogate? Could the surrogate, for example, be restricted to a certain weekly intake of alcohol or be prohibited from smoking? Could the surrogate be made to undergo amniocentesis, so as to monitor fetal abnormalities? Could the couple require that the surrogate undergo an abortion if there was unequivocal evidence of fetal deformity?

What if a defective child is born? Would the surrogate be held to be negligent and liable for the extraordinary medical costs incurred on behalf of the child? What if the surrogate refused to release the child to its genetic parents? If the couple no longer wished to be parents, could the surrogate have the first right to adopt the child? Finally, could the surrogate under any circumstances be compelled to provide care for the child? At present, there are no firm responses to these ethical questions.[16]

---

[16]At this writing, 13 states have tried, but failed, to enact laws concerning surrogate parenting. In 1983, the American College of Obstetricians and Gynecologists placed on record its stern reservations about surrogate mothering. Typically, the surrogate mother receives $10,000 to $15,000 for bearing a child. Couples turning to surrogates generally are in their late thirties, have been married for more than 10 years, and have given up on the idea of conventional adoption.

EPILOGUE

The last two decades have seen a surge of medical knowledge and technological advances that few could have foreseen or dared to prophesy. Equally, we can be sure that the next two decades will contain surprises that promise to continue to strain our cultural and moral fabrics. Future medical advances will doubtlessly create thorny problems for which our present ethical concepts do not prepare us. This evinces either a tragic sense of despair that humans can become lost in their own machinations, or a sober, if not optimistic, realization that humans have the capabilities to manage constructively their own destiny.

INDEX

THE SESQUICENTENNIAL SERIES

In its 150 years, Mercer University has pursued the objectives of excellent teaching and superior scholarship by fostering research in a community dedicated to fresh, original thought. As the University celebrates 150 years of academic leadership, one recognition of this milestone is the publication of the Mercer Sesquicentennial Monograph Series by Mercer University Press.

These three volumes, authored by Mercer faculty members, demonstrate the depth and breadth of the school's dedication to its objectives. Focusing on "excellence in scholarship," the Sesquicentennial Series is another example of the University's commitment to research, scholarship, and publication.

In *Patient in the Womb* Professor E. Peter Volpe presents the realities of the malformed child born into today's society, including the effects on family, institutions, government, and, ultimately, on the infant as an individual. Because of tremendous advances in medical technology and the ability to save infants who, in another era, would have died, modern medicine and modern society are confronted by troublesome ethical dilemmas.

E. Peter Volpe is professor of basic medical sciences (human genetics) at Mercer University School of Medicine. A graduate of the City College of New York, Professor Volpe earned the Ph.D. degree in Zoology from Columbia University. Before coming to Mercer, Professor Volpe was Professor of Biology at Tulane University. He is the author of four previous books relating biology and medicine to human concerns. This is his first book for Mercer University Press.